Walter Reuther

LIVES of the LEFT is a series of original biographies of leading figures in the European and North American socialist and labour movements. Short, lively and accessible, they are welcomed by students of history and politics and by everyone interested in the development of the Left.

general editor David Howell

Walter Reuther

Anthony Carew

MANCHESTER UNIVERSITY PRESS

Manchester and New York

distributed exclusively in the USA and Canada by St. Martin's Press

Copyright © Anthony Carew 1993

Published by Manchester University Press
Oxford Road, Manchester M13 9PL, UK

Distributed exclusively in the USA and Canada
by St. Martin's Press, Inc.,
175 Fifth Avenue, New York, NY 10010, USA

British Library Cataloguing-in-Publication Data
A catalogue record for this book is available from the British Library

Library of Congress Cataloging in Publication Data applied for

ISBN 0 7190 2188 4 *hardback*

TO MY FELLOW MEMBERS
OF UAW LOCAL 2138,
BLACK LAKE, MICHIGAN

Printed in Great Britain
by Bookcraft (Bath) Ltd.

Contents

Acknowledgements

This volume is the product of research carried out while holding a Rockefeller Fellowship at the Walter P. Reuther Archives of Labor and Urban Affairs, Wayne State University, Detroit. I am grateful to the Rockefeller Foundation Humanities Fellowship Program for their generous financial support. The subsequent award by the Reuther Archives of a Henry Kaiser travel grant enabled me to complete the research. During my period in Detroit, I was greatly assisted by a number of friends and colleagues attached to the Reuther Archives and the United Automobile Workers. In particular, I wish to thank Dr Philip Mason, Director of the Archives, and his staff, and also Jane Murphey, Librarian in the Research Department of the UAW.

I am indebted to the following people who gave me interviews: Victor Reuther, the late Fania Reuther, Leonard Woodcock, Douglas Fraser, Irving Bluestone, Joseph Rauh, Frank Winn, the late Bill Kemsley, Ruth Weinberg, Dan Benedict, Ethel Polk, George Schermer and Jack Zeller. Several people read the manuscript in draft, and their helpful comments and suggestions have greatly improved the text. I am deeply grateful to the series editor, David Howell, to Joan Keating, Walter Kendall, Laurie Townsend, Mildred Jeffrey, and especially to Jonathan Williams.

Manchester, September 1992

Note on spelling

Throughout the text, the standard English spelling of labour is used except in reference to American labor institutions and in quotations from American sources.

Abbreviations

AALC	African–American Labor Centre
ACTU	Association of Catholic Trade Unionists
ACW	Amalgamated Clothing Workers
ADA	Americans for Democratic Action
AEU	Amalgamated Engineering Union
AFL	American Federation of Labor
AID	Agency for International Development
AIFLD	American Institute for Free Labor Development
ALA	Alliance for Labor Action
CFDT	Confédération Française Democratique du Travail
CFTC	Confédération Française des Travailleurs Chrétiens
CIA	Central Intelligence Agency
CIO	Congress of Industrial Organizations
CPO	Communist Party Opposition (Lovestoneites)
CP (USA)	Communist Party of the USA
DRUM	Dodge Revolutionary Union Movement
FBI	Federal Bureau of Investigation
FE	Farm Equipment Union
FLP	Farmer-Labor Party
FTUC	Free Trade Union Committee (AFL)
ICFTU	International Confederation of Free Trade Unions
I.G. Metall	German Metalworkers Union
IMF	International Metalworkers' Federation
INTUC	Indian Trades Union Congress
IUD	Industrial Union Department (AFL–CIO)
LID	League for Industrial Democracy
NAACP	National Association for the Advancement of Colored People
PCA	Progressive Citizens of America
PSI	Italian Socialist Party
SDS	Students for a Democratic Society
SNCC	Student Nonviolent Co-ordinating Committee
SPD	German Social-Democratic Party
STEP	Social, Technical and Educational Program
TUC	Trades Union Congress
T & GWU	Transport and General Workers' Union
UAW	United Automobile Workers
UE	United Electrical Workers
WFTU	World Federation of Trade Unions
WLB	War Labor Board
YPSL	Young People's Socialist League

Thank heaven for Walter, the Man with a Plan,
A plan on behalf of the laboring man;
A plan for the aged, a plan for the weak,
A plan for the jobless, a plan for the meek,
A plan for employment, a plan for world peace,
May the plans of the Man with a Plan never cease.   Joe Glazer

The "Babe" is Ruth;
but "Walter" 's Reuther.   Ogden Nash

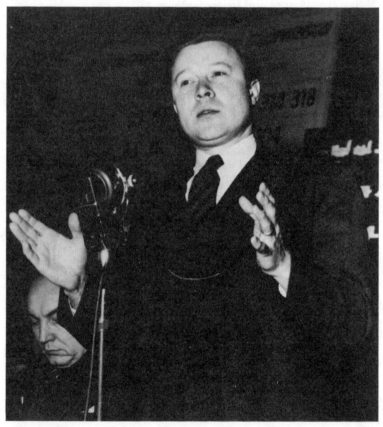

Walter Reuther, Director of the UAW General Motors Department, debating with
General Motors President C.E. Wilson the feasibility of converting automobile
plants to war material production – 31 March 1942. Reproduced by kind permis-
sion of The Archives of Labor and Urban Affairs, Wayne State University

1 From Wheeling to Gorki

Family background is a powerful force. Some transcend their roots, but early conditioning remains an important factor for many. That was especially so of Walter Reuther. Born on 1 September 1907, he was a first-generation American, the son of German immigrants. His father's family were Lutherans from the Rhineland. Part of a religious minority in a predominantly Catholic area, they also lived uncomfortably close to France in a period of Franco-Prussian hostility. Walter's grandfather, Jacob Reuther, a fiercely independent dairy farmer of pacifist views, was unwilling to see his sons conscripted into the Prussian army, and he emigrated to the USA in 1892. His youngest son Valentine, Walter's father, was then 11 years old.

The Reuthers settled on a dairy farm in Effingham, Illinois. A dissident in religious matters, Jacob had difficulty coming to terms with the preaching of the local Lutheran ministers: their concerns were insufficiently related to the problems of the human condition. Eventually he took to conducting his own religious services at home in the log cabin he had built for his family, raising his sons in what is best described as a Christian Socialist environment.

From this rural family background, the 18-year-old Valentine Reuther moved in 1899 to the Ohio Valley town of Wheeling in West Virginia, an industrial centre of steel and glass manufacturing and shipbuilding. Initially he found work in a steel mill and acquired his first experience of trade unionism as a member of the Association of Iron, Steel and Tin Workers. But a strike that he joined ended in the defeat of the union and the loss of his job.

His next employment was as a teamster driving a beer wagon for a German brewery, a job that he held for the next decade. There he helped form a branch of the Brewery Workers' Union and was soon active in the Ohio Valley Trades and Labor Federation, becoming its president at the age of 23. The Federation was to be a major focus of his activity in the years ahead. Through it, he became involved in the affairs of other unions and especially the coal miners' union, on whose behalf he lobbied for improved conditions in the West Virginia state legislature. As a result of his union work, Val Reuther was drawn increasingly into radical politics. He was greatly influenced by Eugene V. Debs, the socialist labour leader and presidential candidate, for whom he campaigned in successive elections, especially among German-speaking workers. He himself ran unsuccessfully as a socialist candidate for the West Virginia state legislature. Prominent in Wheeling community politics, as a former steel trade unionist he led a successful campaign against the town accepting 'tainted' money from steel magnate Andrew Carnegie to build a public library: twelve years earlier Carnegie had been responsible for the brutal crushing of the famous 1892 strike at the Homestead steel mill in Pennsylvania.

In the same year that he became president of the Labor Federation, Val Reuther married Anna Stocker, a recent immigrant from rural Swabia in southern Germany. They settled on Jacob Street in the grimy, working-class district of South Wheeling, a neighbourhood consisting of Poles, Swedes, Yugoslavs and Irish, as well as Germans. Their house was surrounded by factories and coal mines on one side and the tracks of the Baltimore and Ohio Railroad on the other. Between 1905 and 1912 Anna Stocker gave birth to four sons: Theodore, Walter, Roy and Victor. A daughter, Christine, was born eleven years later.

The Reuther brothers were close-knit and strongly influenced by their parents. Both religion and politics were very important in a family that practised the virtues of rural frugality and celebrated the cultural values of the emigré German community. The house contained books, and the children were encouraged to emulate their father's commitment to self-improvement. Walter and his brothers could hardly fail to be influenced by Val's work in the labour movement. 'I take no credit in a personal sense for the fact that I am a trade unionist,' Reuther told the CIO Convention in 1952. 'I was raised in a trade union family . . . Along with my brothers at my father's knee, we learned the philosophy of trade unionism, we got the struggles, the hopes, and aspirations of working people every day.'' On more than one occasion in later years when Walter Reuther was a union president, he brought his father to the platform at conventions and invited him to address the delegation as an old-time union leader. Val Reuther was a friend of Eugene Debs, and when Debs was imprisoned in

Moundsville Penitentiary just south of Wheeling during and after the Great War for his anti-war stance, Val visited him on a number of occasions, and once in 1919 took with him 12-year-old Walter and the youngest son Victor to meet Debs. (Many years later Victor was responsible for restoring Debs's old home in Terre Haute, Indiana and turning it into a museum.)

Opposed to militarism by upbringing, Val strongly supported Debs's position that the war against Germany was dangerous for democracy. As wartime anti-German sentiment ran high, the Reuther home was defaced, hate mail was delivered to the family, and German cultural activities in the town were suspended, including performances by the German choir of which Val was a member. They were very much a German family: Mrs Reuther was addressed as *Mutterschen* while Val was *Vater*; and although Walter was not brought up to speak German and was essentially an all-American boy from the Mid-West, when he visited Berlin in 1959 to address a huge May Day rally at the Brandenberg gate, there was a sense of a son coming home.

Like his father, Val Reuther was inclined to question the teaching of the Lutheran church, and after a violent disagreement with the pastor over the virtues of trade unionism, he ceased attending services while Walter was still at school and lapsed into agnosticism. However, Anna continued to practise her religion devoutly and made sure that Walter and his brothers attended church. Val accepted this, but on Sundays after church would quiz his sons as to what the sermon had been about and would then offer his own views. He encouraged the boys to think about and discuss moral and social questions, and began to assign them debating topics for sessions that were to become a routine part of the Reuther family Sunday. The oratorical skills and sharpness in debate, which Walter and his brothers demonstrated in later life, were attributed in no small part to this practice at home.

Though not as poor as some families in their working-class community, the Reuthers experienced mixed fortunes. Before World War I they were in a position to build a new house in the same South Wheeling district. But soon afterwards, when Walter was only 7, Val Reuther lost his brewery job following the introduction of prohibition in West Virginia. Lacking a skill, he was unemployed for a considerable period during which the family were dependent on income from boarders and an unsuccessful attempt to run a small eating house. Hardship was borne with resourcefulness: Anna Reuther's economies included manufacturing her own soap and making underwear for the family out of flour sacks stitched together. When Val lost an eye in an accident and had to give up his job as a labourer on highway maintenance, he became deeply depressed, and Walter's older brother, Theodore, began working part-time from the age of 11 to supplement the family income. Their fortunes revived when Val eventually secured a position as a life-insurance salesman in the South Wheeling neighbourhood. Even so, Walter decided at the age of 16 to drop out of high school and in 1923 went to work for the Wheeling Corrugating Company, following in Theodore's footsteps.

With two sons working, the financial situation at home improved. In 1926 the Reuthers moved out of Wheeling into a rambling old farmhouse on Bethlehem Hill which they renovated themselves. The move was part of a search for a more salubrious atmosphere for Anna Reuther who had been in poor health. The pull of the countryside was still strong, even if it meant at first living in a harsher environment. From that point on this was to be the family home, to which the Reuther sons would later return occasionally to visit their parents. Val and Anna Reuther enjoyed long lives, Val dying less than three years before Walter, while Anna survived her famous second son.

It was from Bethlehem Hill that Walter Reuther left for Detroit at the age of 19. 5 feet 8 inches tall, of stocky build, with an oval-shaped, freckled face and his mother's red hair, he looked, in his own words, like a 'farmer boy'. With a natural aptitude for mechanics, he had learned fast during his three years as an apprentice toolmaker at the Wheeling Corrugating Company. There he had been earning 42 cents an hour, but now he was anxious for a bigger challenge and was confident that he could handle it.

Detroit, the centre of the growing automobile industry, was a prosperous town in the lush years of the 1920s. It was a magnet for all sorts of workers in search of high wages, and housing and office construction boomed. In 1929 slightly more than 470,000 worked in its auto factories, a large percentage of them from the southern states – Arkansas hillbillies, Kentucky farmers, mountain men from Tennessee, and Alabama cotton pickers. In the late 1920s Ford was retooling to produce the new Model A, and skilled workers were in big demand to build and install 15,000 new machines and retool 25,000 others.

On 27 February 1927 Reuther travelled up to Detroit with Leo Hores, a man some six years his senior with whom he had worked at the corrugating plant in Wheeling. They stayed one night with a friend of Val Reuther's, but then found accommodation in a rooming house. The next day they were hired on the night shift at Briggs Body Works in Highland Park, Reuther working thirteen-hour shifts as a drill press operator at 70–75 cents an hour. He remained for three weeks and then moved to a better job on the day shift at the Ford Highland Park plant. There he was employed as a die maker – precision work on car body presses – starting at $1.05 an hour at a time when average earnings in manufacturing industry were 54 cents. Some months later, as tool room operations ceased at Highland Park, Reuther was transferred to the big River Rouge plant in Dearborn where, as a die leader, he took charge of a group of men during the next three years.[2] At the Rouge plant his pay rose to $1.45, making him very much a labour aristocrat.

Conscious that his formal education was incomplete, Reuther was determined to finish his schooling and perhaps go further, as he entertained hopes of becoming an engineer. He enrolled at Fordson High School in 1928 and set himself the demanding task of completing his education while working on the second shift at Ford. In a hectic routine, he would spend mornings in school, grab a hurried lunch and then turn up at work on a shift that saw him arrive back in his lodgings at bed time. In these years he drove himself hard and demonstrated the sort of tenacity and will power that was to be the hallmark of his trade union career. His determination that every second should count towards some positive goal is captured in an essay on 'Time' that he wrote for Fordson High on 24 October 1929:
'In our lives, the thing that really counts is not how long we live, nor how hard we work, but what we accomplish. Time is one of the greatest factors in our efforts to accomplish our aims; therefore

By wasting of your Time,
You do yourself the greatest crime.'[3]

His essays also reveal a fascination with famous populist and democratic leaders in history. One on Thomas Paine was entitled 'The misunderstood hero', while another, written in November 1929, compared the lives of Napoleon and Lincoln. The essay reveals the rhetorical style, the worthy sentiments, the optimism and eager self-confidence that were to be part of his life as a union leader. It could have been a text for the way he later viewed his own role:

> Lincoln gained power that he might serve humanity, Napoleon gained power that he might rule humanity ... I often think of the wonderful accomplishments that would have been possible with the manpower and wealth wasted by Napoleon for personal honor ... What a wonderful world this would be if all the leaders in the chain of history ... had been inspired with noble ideals to uplift and to serve humanity instead of ruling. Time is fast changing our conception of greatness ... Today [it is] judged from the fruitfulness of a man's life, his accomplishments, and service to humanity ... men like Lincoln shine forth to guide us along the path of justice and equality.[4]

But for the time being, the notion of service to humanity was mere dreaming. There is no evidence from his first two years in Detroit of any involvement in the labour movement. He recorded on his YMCA membership application form that his ambition was to become a labour leader; but that was given only as a second choice, the first being chicken farmer.[5] Detroit was then an 'open shop' town and, like his fellow workers, Reuther did not belong to a union.

With the Wall Street collapse of 1929, the fortunes of the automobile industry plummeted, but Reuther kept his job through the worst years of the Depression. He was earning high wages, and though he sent money home regularly for the first two years, his father refused to accept any more from him after he had turned 21. Single, well-paid and with no major commitments, Reuther was even in a position to invest the princely sum of $2,400 in three plots of building land in nearby Dearborn for speculative purposes. Where his life was heading at this time can only be a matter for conjecture. A colleague from those days, Merlin Bishop, observed that it was only in 1930, when Reuther was joined in Detroit by his younger brother Victor, that radical politics became a serious preoccupation. Victor had dropped out of a university course after his first year, disillusioned by the frivolous, middle-class mentality of his fellow students, and in coming to live with Walter in Detroit, the intention was that they would study jointly at the City College of Detroit (later Wayne State University) now that Walter had graduated from high school.

In 1930 they rented a basement apartment along with three of Walter's friends who, like him, were working their way through college, and the two brothers registered for courses in economics and sociology at the City College. Self-confident and assertive, Walter Reuther had never been short of leadership qualities; at Fordson High he had helped found and then become president of a student club dedicated to promoting social and charitable activities among mature students. But now at the City College his leadership qualities began to assume a political hue. With Victor, he founded the Social Problems Club, an explicitly political organisation affiliated to the socialist League for Industrial Democracy. This was, in effect, the campus young socialist group and the club brought to the student community socialist speakers such as Norman Thomas, Scott Nearing and Harry Laidler. Members encouraged each other in the reading of socialist and radical literature while at the same time campaigning against segregated swimming facilities and compulsory military training for students. In an early clash with communist students, this Reuther-led organisation also thwarted an attempt by members of the Communist Party to reorganise a chapter of the National Student League at the college.[6]

In company with Victor, Walter now seems to have embarked on a journey of social discovery in Detroit. While they studied the social sciences, the two also explored the living examples of poverty and deprivation in the working-class communities around them. Once they spent a weekend in a Salvation Army flophouse in order to experience for themselves the living conditions of the homeless. In the summer of 1932 they were joined in Detroit by their brother Roy, recently laid off from his electrician's job in Wheeling, and they now rented an apartment on Merrick Avenue near the City College where the three of them attended classes. Political activities became more serious in this presidential election year, and during the summer Walter and Victor toured the towns of Michigan in Walter's car, speaking and campaigning on behalf of Norman Thomas's bid for the presidency as a socialist candidate.

As the Depression deepened, employment in the Detroit automobile industry almost halved between 1929 and 1931. It was barren territory for trade unions and yet there was a growing need for collective organisation as unemployment swung the balance of advantage still more decisively in favour of the employers. On the shop floor the foreman was all-powerful. Ford's methods of production treated workers like factors of production, and a rigid system of factory discipline kept workers subservient. Even several years later Herbert Harris was able to write:

motor car manufacturers still lack toward their workers even that rudimentary sense of responsibility which prompts any dirt farmer to pasture a faithful horse; they remain indifferent to how fast the men wear out as long as there are others to replace them . . . When the shift is over the workers tumble half-dead with fatigue into buses, trolleys, or their own cars . . . Some acquire nervous twitchings popularly called 'the shakes'. They get home too tired to do anything but eat and go to bed.[7]

Toolroom workers were less affected by the system of speed-up of work than were production workers, and the effect was that many of Reuther's workmates regarded themselves as an elite group. Nevertheless, Reuther found himself suddenly laid off from the Ford plant in November 1932 without any formal explanation. He assumed that the Ford Service Department's system of spying on employees had alerted them to his political leanings and that he was being victimised for his socialist campaigning during the recently-concluded presidential election, some of which had been carried out in the Ford-controlled town of Dearborn.

He treated his dismissal as if it was a release, and soon decided with Victor to take this opportunity of freedom from employment to see something of the world. Ford had recently concluded an agreement with the Soviet trading company, Amtorg, to sell tools and dies for manufacturing a Soviet version of the Model A which was to be assembled at a new plant in Nizhni Novgorod. A number of Ford workers had gone to the USSR to help train Soviet workers in the use of this equipment, and through one of these, John Rushton, who was a friend, Walter secured a training post with Amtorg. His skills were sufficiently in demand that he even managed to induce Amtorg to offer Victor work as well, though his brother had no training. The Reuthers' plan was to take an extended trip around Europe before moving on to work in what had been named the Molotov plant. They were to sail from New York in mid-February 1933.

Ironically, as they were making preparations for the European trip the climate for trade unionism in Detroit began to improve. Roosevelt had been elected in November and the depressed auto industry began to revive in the winter of 1932 and early 1933. Renewed attempts to organise the industry's workers began, involving craftworkers such as toolmakers, and frequently led by communists, whose Auto Workers Union had existed for some years as a frail organisation. The first stirring was at Briggs where a strike started on 23 January 1933 over a pay cut. The Reuthers and other members of the Social Problems Club joined the Briggs picket line in solidarity as the strike spread to other plants and 15,000 workers came out. Since Briggs was also a supplier to Ford, a large section of Detroit's automobile production was affected. It was the biggest industrial action ever seen in the city, and though the strike eventually collapsed in March, it was the first of several that erupted in Detroit over the next couple of years.

Victor Reuther recalls that he and Walter took their leave of brother Roy at the Briggs picket line as they left Detroit to prepare for their European trip. They spent a few days in New York, staying one night with Norman Thomas who had been their invited speaker at the Social Problems Club. Before they set sail Walter completed an article on the Briggs strike that he had been writing for the *Student Outlook*. In this factual account of the strike, he demonstrated an awareness of the history of autoworker unionism and clear support for the industrial form of unionisation pioneered by the Industrial Workers of the World and later reflected in the structure of the Auto Workers Union.[8]

The Reuthers sailed on the SS *Deutschland* on 16 February and arrived in Hamburg on 24 February, just three days before the Reichstag fire. It was an eventful time to be in Germany: Hitler had been appointed Chancellor on 30 January and the Nazis were about to take power. Walter and Victor made for Berlin where they had a letter of introduction from Norman Thomas to a socialist student group. They stayed for a few days in this student co-operative, seeing at first hand the evidence of Nazi activity in crushing left-wing opposition until, on 5 March, immediately following the Nazi election victory, the co-operative was raided by storm troopers. Some of their student hosts now prepared to leave the country or go underground.

Walter and Victor moved on by way of Dresden and Nuremberg to Swabia where their mother's brothers still lived, planning to make this their European base. The influence of Nazism was evident within their own family, with their uncles divided over the issue and one already a supporter of Hitler. They were alarmed by the atmosphere in Germany, and in late March 1933 were happy to leave the country on a two-month cycling tour. This was to take them into southern France, Italy, Austria and Switzerland, and they hoped that by the time they returned to Swabia the papers permitting them to work in the Soviet Union would have arrived. In the course of their travels they witnessed the increasing hold of fascism and the growing number of swastikas in

9

parts of Europe, and were deeply depressed by what they saw.

Since their papers for the Soviet Union had still not arrived when they returned to Swabia, they set out again in June on another leg of their European cycling tour, travelling now through the Rhineland, to France and then across to Britain. This time they combined labour movement events and car factory visits with their general sightseeing. In Cologne they saw the Ford plant, in France they visited the Citroën plant and then extended their stay in Paris to visit the August conference of the Socialist International where they encountered figures such as the exiled Italian socialist, Pietro Nenni, with whom, many years later, they would have important dealings. Travelling on to Britain, they had a letter of introduction to Fenner Brockway, a prominent member of the Independent Labour Party and former Member of Parliament who arranged for them to visit the conference of the Trades Union Congress (TUC) in Brighton. They also attended the Labour Party conference in nearby Hastings. At the TUC they were introduced to Jennie Lee, the future Member of Parliament and wife of Aneurin Bevan who also became a friend of Walter Reuther. These were contacts that the Reuthers would use to good effect in future years. Indeed, the whole trip to Europe, coinciding as it did with significant political developments on the Continent, invested the brothers with an air of great worldly experience on their return to the United States. They were 'men of affairs' who had rubbed shoulders with some important names and had been present at significant events. Before concluding their visit to Britain which took them to Birmingham, the Potteries and Merseyside, they squeezed in visits to the Morris car plant at Cowley and the Austin works at Longbridge.

In late October 1933, Walter and Victor returned to Germany via The Netherlands where they renewed contact with Emil Gross, the Berlin student leader with whom they had stayed briefly seven months earlier and who was now organising an underground network in Germany. They agreed to take information to one of his contacts in Dortmund, an activity that carried with it a certain danger, though it would provide extra spice when the saga of the European trip was recounted in future years. At length, with their travel papers approved, they left Swabia in November for the USSR.

A three-day rail journey from Berlin brought them to Gorki, the new industrial centre 250 miles north-east of Moscow and half-a-dozen miles from the Volga town of Nizhni Novgorod. At the Molotov automobile factory where they were to work for the next eighteen months, they were housed in a special compound for American technicians who were helping to install the plant. Walter's job was to train a team of workers, many of them peasants, in toolroom operations. Although the Americans had their own restaurant and shopping facilities, the Reuthers chose to take their meals with the Soviet workers. For some months conditions were rather spartan, but they were enthusiastic participants in the creation of this new workers' state. Walter wrote letters to the English-language *Moscow Daily News* commenting on the great spirit of the workforce and making suggestions for improving efficiency and safety. He and Victor were officially invited guests at the 1934 May Day parade in Moscow.[9]

Although Victor's memoir, written forty years afterwards, suggests that he and Walter were conscious of the growing Stalinist repression that led up to the great purges, their joint letters written home at the time conveyed no sense of criticism of the Soviet system. In testimony in 1958 to a US Senate Committee investigating union malpractice, Victor recalled that

> some of my letters conveyed my initial sense of enthusiasm over my personal participation in the vast efforts that the Russian people were making . . . If I was carried away by the experience of the first few months to the point of making this seem more important than the general trend of the Russian dictatorship, I was never carried away far enough to become, myself, a Communist.[10]

Yet there is no doubt that both Walter and Victor Reuther were, like many well-wishing visitors to the Soviet Union in the 1930s, very impressed by what they had seen. Criticism was something that came only after the event. They wrote jointly to Detroit labour lawyer Maurice Sugar in June 1935, having completed their stint at the Gorki factory and about to commence a sightseeing tour of the USSR: 'The shop life here with the Red Corner and the multiplicity of social and cultural activities, the atmosphere of freedom and security . . . make an inspiring contrast to what we know as Ford Wage Slaves in Detroit.'[11]

For five months from late 1934 to the summer of 1935, Walter had lived in a common law relationship with a Russian woman, evidently his first romantic attachment. It was a harmless affair, though he seems to have maintained some contact with her through John Rushton after leaving the USSR. But the relationship would come back to haunt him more than twenty years later when, in an attempt to discredit him, the Soviet newspaper *Trud* stated that he had been legally married to the woman before abandoning her. The paper's claim was that Reuther was a bigamist.

The Reuthers had been relatively well paid in Gorki, and since one of the privileges of foreign workers was ease of movement within the country, they took the opportunity to travel extensively in the USSR in the summer of 1935 after their work was finished. This time their peregrinations by rail took them to the Ukraine, the Black Sea, Georgia, Samarkand and Tashkent, through Central Asia to Peking and Shanghai and finally to Japan where they again hired bicycles in Osaka and toured the country until their money ran out. They worked their passage back to the United States on the SS *Hoover*, arriving in Los Angeles in October 1935, two-and-a-half years after their departure.

Biographers of famous figures at times will look for evidence in the early life of their subject to suggest the inevitability of their subsequent rise to prominence. Walter Reuther has often been written about in this vein. His brother Victor's memoir leaves the impression that much of Walter's early manhood was a conscious preparation for his later mission in life. Accordingly, from 1930 when the two of them registered in the social studies programme at the City College and embarked on their student political activities, until 1935 when they returned from work and travel abroad, they were seeking theoretical principles and practical experience to equip them for leadership in the labour movement. Walter's romantic dalliance in Gorki threatened to upset this project for, as Victor says, they had forsworn marriage so as not to be encumbered in a life's work that they anticipated would be hard.[12] Walter Reuther subsequently demonstrated a single-minded pursuit of trade union leadership and that does make it tempting to see his whole adult life in terms of his 'irresistible rise'. But such accounts have more to do with iconography than reality.

What can fairly be said is that, coming from the socialist and labour background in which he was reared, it was not surprising that Walter Reuther grew up believing in the values of the labour movement. Given his father's tutoring and forceful example, Reuther's quest for self-improvement, his attraction to moral notions of equity and justice, his appetite for debate and, above all, his absolute sense of self-confidence are easily understood. Yet in his early twenties it seems possible that he could have gone on to become a successful engineer; given his energy and determination, it is hard to conceive of him not being successful. His brother's companionship in Detroit from 1930 seems to have been the factor that concentrated his mind on politics. Being dismissed from Ford and then having the time and the where-withal to tour and work in Europe and the USSR were fortuitous events. But in seizing wholeheartedly this opportunity to broaden his horizons, Reuther showed remarkable drive and resourcefulness. Travel abroad seems to have crystallised his determination to work in and for the labour movement in the United States. But what made this feasible was that the world had moved on since 1933. The automobile industry was now ripe for unionisation.

2 Building the autoworkers' union

After the walkout at Briggs in 1933, an official in the mayor's office in Detroit noted that other strikes 'just burst like lightning on the Detroit scene'.[1] But the most significant auto strike in the next eighteen months was at the Auto Lite plant in Toledo, Ohio, in which strikers clashed with the National Guard, tear gas was used and two demonstrators were killed, with scores more wounded. The episode led to some gains but, more importantly, it blooded a group of leaders who would play a significant role in the labour movement in the years to come. Following this event, one sympathetic observer wrote with some prescience: 'nothing can stop the success of unionism in the auto industry . . . There will be more strikes . . . all of them will be like dress rehearsals for the Big Drama to come – when the workers tackle the General Motors citadel in Flint.'[2] Flint in southern Michigan was the hub of the General Motors (GM) empire, and a confrontation there was still more than two years away. In the autumn of 1934 Walter Reuther's brother Roy took a job in adult education with the Flint Board of Education. He wrote that there were great opportunities for union organisation, and in the months ahead he played a major part in preparing the ground for what was to come in 1937.[3]

Attempts at unionisation in the auto industry had been bedevilled by the American Federation of Labor's (AFL) historic conservatism and commitment to the craft principle of union organisation. The more vigorous efforts at organising workers had come from independent union groups, but these were small and lacked resources. With Roosevelt's New Deal legislation seeming to extend to workers the right to belong to a union and bargain collectively, the AFL were increasingly under pressure to adopt a more systematic approach to recruitment, and there was strong support among autoworkers for unionisation to take place on an industrial basis. Acceding to this pressure, the AFL chartered a new union, the United Automobile Workers, in August 1935. Yet the organisation was not initially self-governing, with leaders freely elected by the membership. The AFL were still not reconciled to the principle of industrial unionism, and this led opponents of the Federation line to create within the AFL a Committee for Industrial Organization, soon to become the independent Congress of Industrial Organizations (CIO).

The CIO was formed by miners' leader John L. Lewis in November 1935, the same month that Walter Reuther returned to Detroit. Reuther tried to find work at the Murray Body Company, but the firm discovered who he was before he started. He then took a job for a couple of months at the Coleman Tool and Die Company, where he worked under an assumed name before being fired for attempting to organise the workers. One of Reuther's first steps on returning to Detroit was to go to see Maurice Sugar, the Communist-sympathising labour lawyer with whom the brothers had corresponded from Gorki. Sugar referred Reuther to William Weinstone, the Communist Party's district organiser in Detroit, as someone who could advise him on useful work that he might do. According to Sugar, Weinstone told Reuther to find a base in a car factory – not a very original suggestion, but their meeting did indicate that Walter was close to the communists.[4] Another indication of where his sympathies lay was that in November 1935 he opened a bank account and at the same time bought USSR 7 per cent Gold Bonds worth $2,434.05 – possibly paid for with money realised from the sale of his building plots. At the time of opening this account, he gave his occupation as 'student'.[5]

From around the end of 1935, Reuther appears to have been without paid employment. He undertook some lecturing to left-wing organisations on his Soviet visit and was an active member of a group of Detroit socialists who were helping to build the UAW. His brother Victor had gone as a student to Brookwood, the labour college established by A. J. Muste in New York State. In January 1936 Tucker Smith, a staff member at Brookwood and a future socialist vice-presidential running-mate of Norman Thomas, offered Walter a field job in Pittsburgh as a labour educator, a post to be created in co-operation with the CIO. Reuther's reply reveals his thinking:

> In view of my background in the auto industry and the present situation in the union set up . . . I had thought I could be more effective by going in as a rank and filer and working my way up. This approach, I am well aware, is a slow and laborious one and would somewhat limit the scope of my activity and it would be some time before I could utilize much of my experience.

These restrictions and limitations, although most regrettable, I felt were part of the price that had to be paid.

I had not thought of going into workers' education . . . but if you think I can contribute more to the movement and better utilise my experience in the field of workers' education I am ready to come along.[6]

The hesitant tone and readiness to defer to another's judgement were not characteristics that would recur too often in the future.

Despite Reuther's preference for working in Detroit, the tentative agreement reached with Smith was that he would fulfil speaking commitments already arranged for February and take up his job towards the end of the month. But growing involvement in union activities was to wreck this scheme. On 13 February 1936 he was inducted into membership of the UAW's Local 86 covering GM's Ternstedt plant and he left Detroit immediately afterwards on a lecture tour of Ohio, evidently torn between the prospect of work for Brookwood and responsibilities to the union in Detroit.

A week later he wrote to Tucker Smith from Akron, Ohio, telling him of his change of heart. He had intended to travel on to Brookwood after delivering his lectures, but since then he had received a letter from Victor and Roy stressing the necessity of his staying in the auto industry. On the road, he had also had a long talk with his friend Merlin Bishop who urged him to return to Detroit and work in the auto union. As he explained in his letter to Smith before leaving home, his 'comrades in the Socialist Party' had expressed the feeling that he was running away from one of the most important fields of trade union work. And having recently returned from a country where the opinion of comrades could not be overlooked, he felt the resentment of his Detroit colleagues very keenly: 'in the face of all this comradely pressure I have decided to return to Detroit and work in the auto union.' Another factor, he explained, was that, as well as recently joining the UAW,

I have been elected as a delegate to the Central Body. Then too there is the convention of the Auto International to be held before April 30 and there is much work to be done by the progressive group in order to mobilize all their forces for the convention. The success of the progressive group at this convention is the paramount question in the auto situation at the present time and I feel I could do considerable work toward the coordination and unification of the progressive elements during the next two months.[7]

The die was now cast, and Walter Reuther was committed to working within the UAW. At the union's founding convention in 1935, the American Federation of Labour (AFL) had placed it under the control of a conservative appointee. Reuther now supported those who were seeking full autonomy from the AFL in order to build a real industrial union. Though unemployed, he was busy that spring working to consolidate the position of the Progressive Caucus, as the anti-AFL group was called. The focus of their activity was the union convention at South Bend, Indiana in April. As he explained to Victor, he was receiving almost daily requests for speaking engagements, but was turning them down because of the pressure of work for the Caucus. One extracurricular activity that he did find time for was his marriage on 13 March to May Wolf, a schoolteacher and active socialist. The event did not rate an entry in his diary, unlike a speaking engagement for the same day. His marriage was clearly an impulsive affair and broke the agreement to remain single that he had made with Victor. Yet Walter and May's partnership was a strong one that passed the test of time.

At the time of the South Bend convention Walter Reuther was clearly conscious that he was taking part in a major historic event which would have far-reaching consequences. In earnest tones, he wrote to Victor about the drama that he was involved in:

> ... we are getting ready for one of the greatest battles in the history of organized labor. Never has organized labor face [sic] such an aggregate of organized capital. It is a mans [sic] job, one that will test the best that is in us but it must be done and I am fortunate to have been elected to a position where I can take a leading part in this historical task of storming the stronghold of the open shop.

He linked this historic moment of the labour movement to his own personal fortunes and described to Victor how he had been caught up in a whirlpool of pressures:

> we had both planed [sic] on approaching the trade union field and the political setup (to say nothing of matters of a more personal nature) with the utmost caution, feeling our way inch by inch ever with our feet firmly on the ground. As usual there was a wide discrepancy between plans and actuality. Caught in the current of a series of ever accelerating and propelling events I was driven forward culminating as it were on the vortex of a whirlpool, stimulated, ready to ride the next crest. Three months ago I was a humble trade unionist now I am an AF of L bureaucrat; three months

ago I was a rank and filler [*sic*] agitating for a Farm Labor Party now I am Vice chairman of the Wayne County FLP ... this is a remarkable age, the zep crossed the Atlantic in 49 hours, nothing is impossible ... I have caught the spirit of the age.[8]

In April he hitched a lift to South Bend for the UAW convention. This was to be the start of his career as a union leader. As a delegate, he was supposed to be employed at the Ternstedt plant. However, on the first day of the convention Reuther had to overcome challenges to his credentials on the grounds that he had not worked at Ternstedt and that he was also a communist. The first point was true, though he told the convention that he had been forced to work under an assumed name. The charge of being a communist was probably unfounded, though the extent of Reuther's links with the Communist Party in this period have never been completely clarified. However, the important point is that the challenge to his credentials served only to build him up from an unknown delegate to a major convention figure. Within the Michigan delegation Reuther established himself as one of the spokesmen and was elected by the state caucus to the union's executive board. At South Bend, the UAW became fully self-governing, with freely chosen officers. Its first elected president was Homer Martin, a former preacher from Kansas City and a man destined to be the focus of a major battle within the union in the next three years.

At the time of the convention, only 30,000 of half a million auto workers were unionised and there was not a single collective agreement in the industry in Michigan, where 70 per cent of the workforce lived. A vigorous recruiting campaign was planned, the intention being to undertake general educational work during the slack summer season and to build up a competent staff, so as to be able to go on the offensive in the autumn when the auto industry would begin to retool its plants for the new model cars. Reuther began to consolidate the organisation in his district – the west side of Detroit – persuading six local unions with a total membership of seventy-eight to amalgamate and to form what was known as the West Side Local with himself as president. In the years ahead, this was to be his union base, and by December 1937 the West Side Local had 30,000 members. The union's treasury was minimal and Reuther personally financed the UAW office on Michigan Avenue and Twenty-Fourth on borrowed money.

The UAW's immediate target was to organise workers at GM whose key plants were in Flint, followed by those at firms supplying parts to Ford in anticipation of a major drive there. Reuther, with his base in the West Side, would not play a central role in the big 1937 organising drive in Flint. However, Kelsey Hayes, the major supplier of brake shoes to Ford, was in his territory, and so was the Ford Rouge plant itself. By late 1936 a number of UAW activists had managed to infiltrate the workforce at Kelsey Hayes; these activists included Victor Reuther, whom Walter had brought to Detroit for the purpose. With Walter Reuther having already arranged a meeting with Kelsey Hayes management for 11 December to discuss grievances related to the speed of production, the core UAW members in the plant called a strike the day before, hoping to apply pressure on management to coincide with the meeting. The stoppage developed into a sit-down strike and lasted five days before a compromise settlement was reached. In one of the first sit-downs, unionism had been established at Kelsey Hayes. Yet a more important citadel was shortly to be stormed in Flint and Reuther needed to settle at Kelsey Hayes in order to free UAW resources for that encounter.[9] And so, as soon as the Kelsey Hayes strike ended, Victor Reuther departed for Flint.

The events surrounding the great sit-down strike at GM's Flint plants, which began on 29 December 1936 and ended forty-four days later with the recognition by management of the UAW, has been thoroughly documented. Walter Reuther was not centrally involved in what was undoubtedly a fierce and at times bloody episode, though his two brothers played a prominent role. Walter's contribution was to support the Flint action by leading a nine-day sit-down strike at the GM Cadillac plant in Detroit starting on 8 January. However, he later took a share of the credit (some would say without justification) for a daring tactical ruse under which the key Chevrolet No. 4 plant at Flint was occupied by strikers, despite being heavily guarded by armed security personnel.[10]

Walter's own moment of physical heroism came three months later in May 1937 during an early attempt to recruit members at the Ford River Rouge plant, in what has come to be known as the Battle of the Overpass. On 26 May Reuther and fellow UAW executive board member Richard Frankensteen attempted to hand out recruiting literature to workers coming off shift and leaving the Ford plant via a highway overpass which was company property. For the union men, it was a calculated exercise to see how far they could go with Ford management. Reuther anticipated trouble and had invited representatives of the Conference of Civil Rights and the Senate Civil Liberties Committee to be present, as well as news reporters and photographers. As they leafleted, Reuther and Frankensteen were assaulted by a number of hired thugs in the pay of the Ford Service Department. The National Labor Relations Board, which investigated the incident following a complaint by the UAW, found Ford guilty of deliberately planning and carrying out the assault. According to the NLRB:

> The story of the attack is almost unbelievably brutal. Reuther and Frankensteen were singled out for particular attention and given a terrific beating. Each of them was knocked down and viciously pounded and kicked in all parts of the body. They were then raised in the air several times and thrown upon their backs on the concrete. Reuther was then kicked down the north stairway and beaten and chased down Miller Road . . .[11]

A number of newspapers and magazines, including *Time*, reported the incident with grim photographs of the two men bruised and bloody. It was a frightening experience but it raised Reuther's profile within the union and it gave early proof of his physical courage, a trait that even his enemies could never deny.

It was ironic that photographs taken after the event showed Reuther and Frankensteen with arms draped around each other's shoulders, for the two would soon be on opposite sides in the bitter factional dispute that was about to break out in the UAW. There were many dimensions to this infighting, but for these two men it concerned the major practical question of who was to be responsible for future organising efforts at Ford.

From its victory in gaining recognition at GM, the UAW had moved on to tackle Chrysler in April in an equally successful seventeen-day sit-down strike. The union was now growing by leaps and bounds: from an organisation of a few thousand members at the start of the year, it was on the way to having 350,000 dues-payers by summer. Militancy was everywhere, and in April Walter Reuther himself led another sit-down at the Yale and Towne key factory, which ended with the workers being evicted and himself arrested. However, the militancy that had been generated by the union's organising drive began to destabilise the UAW itself. The Chrysler strike was followed by continued unofficial action, and at GM, too, there were 170 strikes between April and June 1937. Divisions now opened up among the leadership of the young union and rivalries emerged that came close to paralysing the organisation in the next two years. In all this, Walter Reuther was a leading participant, and the period was a significant landmark in his political and trade union development.

The factional disputes were coloured by personal jealousies in circumstances where the UAW president, Homer Martin, was a weak and erratic figure and where would-be successors, of whom Reuther was certainly one, were keen to demonstrate their competence as leaders. It involved political differences in that rival groups drew support from followers of different political parties among the UAW membership. Most of all, however, the conflict turned on rival concepts of how a union should be organised and led. Indeed, it reflected deep differences about how to maintain a union as a stable organisation without sacrificing its essential militancy. Unfortunately, the dispute was so vigorous that the union came close to fragmenting before the conflict was settled.

The differences emerged after the Chrysler strike, when Martin accused communists in the union of fomenting wildcat strikes. Throughout the fighting, partisans were identified as pro-Martin or anti-Martin, though some changed allegiances and others at times sat on the fence. At root it was a conflict between on the one hand those who took their lead from communists, and on the other Martin loyalists aided by the Communist Party Opposition (CPO), that is, supporters of Jay Lovestone, the former general secretary of the CP(USA) who had fought with Stalin in the late 1920s, had been expelled from the Comintern and was now bitterly anti-Stalinist. Aligned with the communists were socialists and members of the Association of Catholic Trade Unionists, while Martin and Lovestone counted on the support of some Trotskyists.

In the face of continued shop-based militancy following the Chrysler strike, Martin turned to Jay Lovestone for assistance in combatting the communists, and a dozen 'Lovestoneites' were appointed to the UAW staff. That there was a genuine problem is reflected in a letter from CIO organiser Adolph Germer to John L. Lewis, written after a visit to Detroit: 'I told them [the UAW leaders] that outside of Detroit . . . every CIO representative is looked upon as a walking strike and that this epidemic is going to make it difficult to organize other industries

. . . I pointed out that it was high time that unauthorized strikes must come to an end; that unless it does their organization will surely go on the rocks . . .'. He also told Martin that he should get rid of both the warring communists and CPO people from his staff, but Martin's aim was to consolidate his position by centralising control in the union and utilising the experience of his CPO allies in fighting the communists.[12]

In this dispute Reuther was drawn in on the side of the communists, so it is important to establish the nature of his political orientation at this time. He had returned from his foreign travels sympathetic to the USSR and disposed to co-operate with communists in the auto industry. He was a member of the Socialist Party but was not one to accept party discipline in every situation and was identified with that group in the Detroit branch who held it to be sectarian not to engage in united front tactics with the communists. There was indeed a flavour of Leninism in the way he viewed political action in 1936. Writing to Victor at the time of the South Bend convention, he described how, as a socialist, he was working with communists to build a Farmer-Labor Party (FLP) and had recently been elected vice-chair of the Wayne County FLP:

> We who realize the need of building a small revolutionary disciplined party with mass influence recoganize [sic] the potentialities of a farm labor movement. By working within such a party, as a disciplined unit, with courage and clarity we can use the mass party as a resovour [sic] from which we can draw the most advanced workers into our revolutionary party. This revolutionary party within the mass party must carry on a relentless struggle against the reformistic policy, which is inevitable with such a mass party, on the one hand going along with them in there [sic] lukewarm inadequate programe [sic] but constantly pointing out the possibility of acchieving [sic] freedom, peace, and security without a complete change in our social system. I sincerely believe that to build a Socialist Party we must first build the FLP, they are as much a part of one another as is sowing and reaping.[13]

Reuther was disciplined by his local Socialist Party group for taking this position, though it was party policy to work within the FLP.

Was he an uncritical ally of the communists, blind to their tendency to shift with the wind? After all, within a year, their policy on the FLP had changed and they were now completely behind Roosevelt's Democrats. Reuther was not so credulous. In his letter to Victor he himself raised the question of whether the FLP was merely a communist-inspired body, answering that that was not the case every-where. His line was essentially the pragmatic one: 'be the FLP prema-ture, CP inspired, reformative, opportunistic, or what, it still IS . . . the SP should get in these organisations and fight for correct pos-ition'.[14]

Among socialists, Reuther was often criticised for being too inti-mate with the communists, and there has always been a question about whether he was perhaps for a time even a secret member of the party. Open and declared membership of the CP among UAW members was very rare, though a larger group were 'associated' with the party and accepted its discipline. Reuther was certainly approached several times to join but, according to Howe and Widick, had refused if it meant submitting to discipline on foreign affairs.[15] Senior communists themselves later disputed the facts. Party leader William Z. Foster claimed that Reuther had applied for membership, but that the appli-cation had been turned down on the grounds of his opportunism.[16] On the other hand, Louis Budenz, a one-time editor of the *Daily Worker*, denied the truth of this, claiming that only just before he had been sent to Detroit by the Politburo to try to recruit Reuther into the Red 'top fraction' in the UAW, but Reuther had flatly refused.[17] However, in the papers of Nat Ganley, the party's leading figure in the UAW in Detroit, correspondence relating to a draft biography of a fellow party member asserts that Reuther was a CP member at large and paid his dues to Ganley. According to Ganley, Reuther agreed to remain in the Socialist Party and bore from within, in agreement with the CP. But Ganley's tantalising advice in the correspondence is that the draft memoirs should be corrected to delete any such reference on the grounds that Reuther would deny membership.[18] Certainly, when the Senate's witch-hunting Dies Committee came to Detroit in 1938 to hear evidence, Reuther vehemently denied that he was or ever had been a member or supporter of the Communist Party. Yet there are Reuther critics who doubt the truth of this and have come to regard both his entry and rapid exit from the Communist Party simply as reflections of his 'free wheeling opportunism'.[19]

However, during the early phase of the UAW's factional dispute, Reuther sided with the communists, while trying to find a formula to resolve the real problem that the union was encountering. In a docu-ment he drafted in July 1937, he expressed the belief that the major difference between the two sides had to do with their respective conception of the task of the union at this point in its development.

> The minority [anti-Martin group] holds . . . that the UAW is still in the process of formation. It is a young union, not yet set organizationally or administratively, that must keep itself flexible and on its toes to meet constantly new and changing problems. It must be alert, enterprising, militant, constantly at its best with structural and administrative forms fluid and easily adapted to the new situations . . . our problems are vastly different from the administrative routine of old established unions like the United Mine Workers and International Ladies Garment Workers . . . We need organisation and adaptation, rather than routine administration and regimentation. We have to rely [on] the discipline of militant loyalty and enterprizing courage, rather than that of long-standing custom and habit.[20]

The Martin faction was intent on establishing a more rigid, centralised structure. Besides this fundamental difference of approach, Reuther noted the mass of petty, personal issues and near-issues, which had no bearing on the fundamental division of policy. Both sides misrepresented the other on the question of spontaneous strikes. Neither side favoured these 'because a union cannot continue if it tolerates such major unauthorised actions as unauthorised strikes'. But given that most such strikes were provoked by the employers anyway, Reuther took the pragmatic view that a flexible approach was necessary in handling them.[21]

As the August 1937 UAW convention in Milwaukee approached, both sides built up their organisational strength. Martin and Frankensteen took the initiative here in organising the Progressive Caucus, arguing for the centralisation of union power and an end to unauthorised strikes. In response, the communists and socialist allies organised the Unity Caucus, which also called for union discipline and an end to wildcat strikes; but they also wanted local autonomy and democracy and a determined organising campaign at Ford, which seemed to have been forgotten amidst the feuding.

Though attached to one of the warring groups, Reuther was unhappy at the damage the conflict would do to the union in its dealings with employers, especially with the UAW about to attempt to negotiate a new agreement with GM. As a representative of the Unity Caucus, Reuther had gone to a meeting of the Martin/Frankensteen group to plead for a common approach:

Unity means unity on top and unity on the bottom – unity along the line. Unity means cutting out all political maneuvring and conniving. Unity means the complete abolition of factional struggle and getting down to the struggle of organizational problems – organising Ford . . . etc. We feel that unity is possible by including in the leadership all constructive forces. There is but one test of leadership – that is, merit, experience and competency.[22]

Here was the expression of a view that was to become the governing rule of the Reuther-led UAW in later years – 'unity in the leadership, solidarity in the ranks'.

For Reuther, that unity needed to be based on local democracy and a self-disciplined militancy:

The first point on our program is the question of democracy . . . We can be more democratic by building a more effective shop steward system, that is, enlarged powers for the shop stewards. We want to give the local unions more democracy. They should have complete democracy in the election of officers. Where the union is large enough it should have some voice in deciding who their organizer shall be . . . on the question of discipline, our caucus goes on record for discipline. This is an army of labor; we cannot march forward unless we have effective discipline.

He recognised that an important element in the dispute was the correct interpretation of the union constitution in a situation where the respective powers of the president and the executive board were not clearly defined:

We are in favor of the General Executive Board making its decisions and that these decisions are binding upon the membership . . . Between meetings of the Executive Board, the president interprets the decisions and speaks in the name of the Board. Only we think that in an organization of 350,000 that the responsibility is so great that it should be shared by the vice-presidents, who should have definite powers . . . Can we not have authority and at the same time give certain power to the vice-presidents?

Finally, he argued for leaders to be chosen on merit, not according to party loyalty.[23]

While Reuther was acting as broker for the Unity Caucus to the Martin supporters, he was also dealing independently with Lovestone, and this was to sow seeds of suspicion about him in the minds of his communist colleagues. According to Lovestone, in the summer of 1937 the CPO were becoming impatient with the erratic and unreliable Martin, and so they turned to Reuther with a view to promoting him for leader. He and Lovestone met at the Woodward Hotel in Detroit and Lovestone put forward a detailed policy programme for running the union. However, while Reuther said he was willing to accept most of it, he baulked at the idea of waging a militant struggle against communist penetration of the union. The two men went their separate ways.[24] This account of the meeting has a ring of truth and fits in with Reuther's public position which was to try to work with all factions. But his dealing with Lovestone bred mistrust among the communist supporters. Interestingly, Homer Martin was to claim later that the communist leaders themselves offered to make a deal with him if only he, as president, would agree to appoint some of their people to organising posts. Yet despite their own wooing of Martin, the communists chose to view Reuther's 'private diplomacy' with Martin's strategist as a particularly reprehensible manoeuvre. Nine years later they would resurrect the episode when, as the president of the union, Reuther was deeply embattled with communist opponents.[25]

At the 1937 Milwaukee convention, a riotous event, the Unity Caucus put forward a slate of candidates for election which contained both Unity and Progressive members, and they endorsed Martin for president. Their programme won the day, beating back Martin's attempt to centralise. He was denied the power to dismiss organisers or to eliminate locally published newspapers. Though Reuther and other Unity Caucus leaders worked hard to smooth over differences with Martin, the setback he suffered at the convention prompted the president to lash out in all directions at his opponents. He now tried to prevent communications between locals of the union, local newspapers were abolished, he blocked public discussion of executive board affairs, secured from the board the power to suspend members without trial, and denied the rank and file the right to ratify bargaining settlements. He also attempted to sideline Reuther by depriving him of important assignments. There was to be a repeat of the leafleting at the Overpass on 11 August, but Martin stopped him from taking part under the threat of expulsion.[26] Frankensteen, a Martin supporter, not Reuther, was to be chairman of the Ford organising committee. In UAW politics this was a very significant move for it was generally thought that whoever succeeded in organising Ford would eventually capture the leadership of the union. Only in late 1937 did Reuther go on to the UAW payroll, and Adolph Germer reported to John L. Lewis that he was afraid that Martin might remove Reuther from Detroit altogether and 'send him to the sticks'. Because Reuther was very popular, Germer judged that such a move would be sure to stir up a hornets' nest.[27]

While the internal fight raged, the economic fortunes of the auto industry slumped: over 300,000 workers were unemployed and UAW membership was reduced by three-quarters from its 1936 peak. The weakening of the union was reflected in dealings with the employers. From late 1937 they frequently tried to avoid dealing with shop stewards. Homer Martin conceded to GM the right to fire wildcat strikers, hoping to get exclusive bargaining rights in return. But the company rejected this and a national conference of shop stewards repudiated Martin. Reuther now favoured resuming the sit-downs to secure recognition of the stewards. The attempted renegotiation of the GM agreement had produced a wholly unsatisfactory outcome, and in the wake of this a major unauthorised strike broke out in Pontiac, Michigan in November. Reuther supported the strike, as did the local communists in Michigan, but the national leadership of the Communist Party denounced their action. At this point senior communists seemed to lose faith in Reuther as a reliable ally, while Reuther in turn was coming to see the impossibility of co-operating with people who could be dictated to from on high.[28]

In the course of the Milwaukee convention, communist suspicions of Reuther had grown, while among socialists in the union there was increasing unease about their communist allies. Yet for the time being both parties viewed Martin as the bigger danger. It was international politics that brought their differences into the open, much to the puzzlement of the union rank and file. Whether to support the policy of collective security in the face of fascism (i.e. solidarity with the USSR) or, in keeping with the mid-westerner's instinct for isolationism, to line up with those demanding a referendum before the USA would declare war was an issue which divided the communists and the socialists. And when it was debated in the UAW executive board in January 1938, Reuther found himself with the socialists supporting the latter position and on the same side as Homer Martin. International policy differences were reinforced by socialist disillusionment with communist positions taken in the Spanish Civil War. These foreign policy considerations were now sufficiently important to the communists for them to abandon any restraint in their opposition to Martin.

Unable to dominate the alliance with Reuther, whose personal ambition was increasingly apparent, they decided to destroy it and look for other friends.

Communist leaders now began to pay court to Frankensteen, on whom they secretly promised to bestow electoral favours. Their public break with the Reuther group came when they failed to line up their votes behind Victor Reuther's candidacy for secretary-treasurer of the Michigan CIO at its April 1938 convention. The Michigan CIO had just been formed and the choice of its secretary-treasurer was a matter of practical and symbolic importance.[29] By abandoning the Reuthers in favour of a Homer Martin supporter for this post, the communists could not have made it clearer that the partnership was over. For Walter Reuther it was a betrayal that he would never forget.

He now began to organise his own independent factional group, made up largely of socialists. It was in the course of a gathering of socialist friends discussing the activities of the communists and the Lovestoneites at his Detroit apartment on La Salle Boulevard in April 1938 that two armed men broke into the apartment, assaulted Reuther and attempted to force him to leave with them. The intruders were driven off and shortly afterwards were arrested and tried, though they were acquitted by a jury. No clear motive for the attack was ever established, though Reuther believed that the men had connections with the Ford Company. For the defence, it was suggested that Reuther had staged the whole episode in an attempt to implicate Homer Martin and gain favourable publicity for himself – a line that his UAW opponents were happy to repeat.[30] From the earliest days, he had no shortage of enemies, and some of them were prepared to go to great lengths to silence him.

Though operating as separate forces, the Reuther and the communist factions still had to contend with the ever-more arbitrary leadership of Homer Martin which was leading the union towards disaster. Martin suspended a number of leading officers of the union who opposed him, so creating the conditions for a split. With the communists disposed to fight the president to a finish, and the employers opportunistically withdrawing from collective agreements, Reuther and his socialist supporters pleaded for internal peace and a turning of attention outwards to the problems in the industry.[31] The CIO's leaders were increasingly drawn into the affairs of the UAW, and Reuther was frequently in touch with John L. Lewis, explaining the ongoing tactical twists as the protracted trial of the suspended officers took place under union procedures in summer 1938. While trying to find a compromise solution, no doubt Reuther was hoping to gain the personal support of Lewis for his own group. But Lewis had little time for socialists and was not enamoured of Reuther, whom he regarded as an ambitious upstart.

Eventually, in early 1939 a desperate Homer Martin attempted to lead the UAW back into the AFL fold, the result being that the UAW was effectively split. Separate conventions of the rival groups were held in March, the anti-Martin forces meeting in Cleveland under the watchful eyes of CIO leaders Philip Murray and Sidney Hillman. The task of the Cleveland convention was to elect a new leadership, re-write the union constitution and start building the organisation again. There were four obvious candidates for the presidency, including Reuther and George Addes, the recently suspended secretary-treasurer, who had held that post since 1936 and had now moved into an alliance with the communists. It is a widely-held view that at this point the communist strength in the union was at a peak and that, had they chosen to install their supporters in leadership positions, they would have been able to do so. In that case, George Addes would most likely have become the new president. But the communists were keen to preserve a positive relationship with the CIO leadership, and they bowed to the preference of Murray and Hillman for someone better placed to unite the union. Consequently the more neutral figure of R. J. Thomas was chosen. With prominent communist supporters declining to run for election to the executive board, the party now relied on influence rather than control, so passing up their best-ever opportunity to assert their dominance.

In the rewritten constitution adopted at Cleveland, the emphasis was on decentralised democracy. The president was stripped of all but administrative authority; members could be expelled only through proceedings started in their own local. Councils were also created for each of the major corporations, to enable the membership to be more involved in collective bargaining, and Reuther secured the leadership of the key bargaining council for GM. It was an outcome that helped Reuther's leadership ambitions, giving him time to build his own support. In the years ahead he never viewed Thomas as anything more than an interim leader.

With the employers taking advantage of the rivalry between the

29

UAW–AFL and the UAW–CIO by refusing to deal with either, and workers being asked to choose sides, it was not clear which faction would triumph or, indeed, whether effective unionism would survive in the industry. In these circumstances, it was a strike led by Walter Reuther that decided the matter. In July 1939 GM was in the process of tooling up for the subsequent year's models. Assembly plants were closing, and anyway the fall in membership among production workers meant that the union could not count on these groups in a battle with the company. Barely 10 per cent of the workforce still remained unionised. However, operating within the newly democratised structure of the UAW–CIO, and capitalising on the continued membership strength among skilled workers, Reuther launched a well-organised strike at twelve key plants where retooling was taking place, thus preventing work on the new models. This imaginative 'strategy strike', as it was called, forced the company to concede after four weeks. The UAW–CIO gained exclusive bargaining rights at most GM plants, and in the subsequent National Labor Relations Board representation election, the union scored a decisive win over Martin's union.

By the end of 1939 the turbulent Martin period that had seen the UAW on a rollercoaster ride was over. The union had barely survived the experience, but was now in a position to begin to build for a stable future. Reuther had contributed significantly to this outcome, arguing persuasively the case for maintaining a balance between decentralisation and organisational cohesion, and between the shop militancy that advanced the general interest and the undisciplined workplace disruption that set worker against worker. With Homer Martin had gone the threat of overcentralisation and arbitrary leadership: a more decentralised but disciplined militancy now characterised the UAW, and for Reuther 'discipline' was always a key word. In these years he had come of age politically, rapidly developing the skills of a nimble labour politician. During the anti-Martin struggle, he had initially been close to the communists, and indeed was willing to risk censure by the Socialist Party for maintaining these contacts. It seems that trade union issues concerned him more than party politics, and his participation in Socialist Party activities waned as his UAW responsibilities increased. Doubtless his ties with the communists reflected a straightforward recognition of the need for worker solidarity. Whether or not he was, for a short time, a secret member of the party is of little importance: the fact is that he certainly operated in their orbit. But Reuther was too much his own man for them, and had his own personal ambitions.

It was this independent style, rather than deep differences of view, that at first caused the communists to become suspicious of him and then hostile. They considered him to be an opportunist, while he was increasingly conscious that opportunism was the defining characteristic of communist trade union activity. It was not a question of one side being more or less militant than the other (the labels 'left' and 'right' were always largely meaningless in this situation), and in the late 1930s communist trade unionists were criticised by socialists for their lack of coherence and at times disruptive and reactionary policies. In this situation, Reuther's socialist upbringing and training provided a ready basis on which to define a distinct position on union issues and to organise a separate group of supporters. Sharp policy differences between socialists and communists were coming to the fore — over the Soviet purges, Spain and isolationism — and these all became part of the battleground between him and his erstwhile allies. In 1937 Reuther had argued for an end to factions, for building bridges between different sections of the membership and subordinating personalities to the interests of the organisation. 'Unity on the top and unity on the bottom' was how he put it, and his belief in teamwork and organisational discipline was certainly genuine. But though Homer Martin had now departed, internal rivalries would ensure that factional politics continued. And in this field Walter Reuther was as vigorous and adept as any of his rivals.

3 The path to union president

From 1940 the war in Europe became a major factor in UAW politics. At the union's 1940 convention, delegates were opposed to American involvement but otherwise supported Roosevelt's defence policies. With the communists hobbled by the Nazi–Soviet Pact and the isolationist strains of the *Daily Worker*'s 'the Yanks are not coming', Walter Reuther supported a resolution branding the Soviet Union as an aggressor and totalitarian state. He also joined in the popular support for Roosevelt in the presidential election later in the year. Reuther was now moving into an important phase of his career, in which he pursued goals in co-operation with the Roosevelt administration, and it is necessary to consider how this development came about.

He had been an active member of the Socialist Party before the South Bend convention in 1936. Once elected to the union's executive board, however, his direct participation in party activities declined. In 1937 he was part of the Labor slate in Detroit that ran unsuccessfully for election to the city council, his one and only bid for public office. But in the eighteen months after South Bend, it seems that he attended at most only a couple of party meetings. Doubtless this could be explained in part by the pressure of union activities. However, in November 1938 the gubernatorial election in Michigan provided a major test of Reuther's commitment to the Socialist Party. Running for re-election was the Democratic Governor, Frank Murphy, whose intervention in the 1937 General Motors sit-down had been beneficial to the UAW. Along with other socialists, Reuther was faced with a choice between support for Murphy and the socialist candidate. It was a situation, not uncommon for union members, where ideology and the requirements of practical trade unionism were in conflict. The Socialist Party in Detroit had two branches, and the one embracing auto workers was inclined to adopt a flexible position, allowing members to vote for the incumbent Democrat. An additional consideration for Reuther was that he had now broken with the communists in the

UAW and in the struggle with them was bidding for the support of CIO leaders John L. Lewis and Sidney Hillman. They, in turn, were disposed to build balances of power within the warring UAW and encouraged the development of Reuther's separate caucus, while insisting as a price that he resign from the Socialist Party in order to support Murphy. To save embarrassment, it was proposed that Reuther should be allowed a 'friendly resignation' from the party, an idea that the leader Norman Thomas would not accept. In consequence, Reuther simply dropped out of the organisation.

Was Reuther right to support Murphy? In the event Murphy lost the election to the Republican challenger, in part a victim of the backlash against sit-downs. In this environment a more radical politics was unlikely to succeed. The socialist candidate fared badly and the party suffered a decline. Indeed, it was already in difficulties in Michigan where it had been squeezed during the years of UAW factionalism by the alliance between the CIO and the communists. It had also suffered as a result of Norman Thomas's support for Homer Martin's anti-war stance: Martin was simply not popular with the UAW membership. Throughout 1939, the party was collapsing; it lacked a functioning national headquarters and branches were becoming defunct. With the looming war in Europe, members were also torn over the policy of isolationism, and in the coming months and years many of Reuther's former socialist colleagues in the union quietly followed him out of the organisation. As a close ally Brendan Sexton put it, most of these people did not so much leave the Socialist Party as drift away. They might have remained if the party had had a more realistic sense of American politics, but by 1940 there was a tremendous working-class feeling for Roosevelt.

People like Walter Reuther now had the job of running a large trade union organisation, an altogether different responsibility from that involved in leading a small socialist group.[1] They ignored at their peril the political sentiments of the rank and file. So when in 1940 John L. Lewis publicly disowned Roosevelt, piqued at not being chosen as his presidential running mate, Reuther, together with Thomas and Frankensteen, met the President and expressed the support of the UAW. Reuther then went on radio to counter Lewis's message: 'The issue,' he announced, 'is wholly and simply: Roosevelt or reaction? American labor will take Roosevelt.'[2]

American defence policies altered the terrain on which labour–

33

management relations were conducted. Stepped-up military production to meet the Lend-Lease agreement with Britain, together with a restrained attitude to strikes (the latter being very much a communist–non-communist issue as the party fanned the flames of industrial militancy during this 'imperialist' phase of war), led labour to seek to further its interests through direct contact with the administration. An early and notable example of this was a widely discussed proposal by Reuther in December 1940 which called for tripartite administration of the arms industry in order to meet more efficiently the pressing need for military aircraft production. Reuther's idea prefigured a more general proposal advanced the following year by John L. Lewis's successor as CIO president, Philip Murray, under which unions would be jointly involved with management and government in the running of industry through industrial councils.

Entitled *500 Planes a Day: A Program for the Utilization of the Auto Industry for Mass production of Defense Planes*, Reuther's scheme was an attempt to answer Roosevelt's call to Congress for 50,000 planes a year. It was prompted by the scandal of unused auto plant capacity in circumstances where employers were hoping to induce government to build them new factories for military production rather than insist on the conversion of existing facilities. It began: 'England's battles, it used to be said, were won on the playing fields of Eton. This plan is put forward in the belief that America's can be won on the assembly lines of Detroit.' The Plan called for a central aviation production board consisting of members from management, government and labour. Under such an administrative arrangement, Reuther argued that output would increase through more efficient use of men and machines.[3] Murray presented the Plan to Roosevelt as a joint CIO–UAW proposal, and the President referred it to his Defense Council. In January 1941 Reuther met Roosevelt at the White House to discuss the scheme.

In a number of respects this was an archetypal Reuther initiative. It was an imaginative scheme, boldly presented with a view to gaining maximum publicity. It was revealing that, while Philip Murray's subsequent industrial council proposal produced little resonance, Reuther's scheme became widely known. He enlisted the help of Eddie Levinson (the leading labour correspondent of the *New York Post*) and I. F. Stone in drafting the scheme. He secured valuable publicity from favourable reviews by Walter Lippman and Dorothy Thompson. The

Plan encapsulated a theme central to his emerging social democratic value system – that rational decision-making in industry required the participation of unions as of right, not in a confrontational role, but as partners of government and management. It was inspired by a detestation of inefficiency. It reflected Reuther's awareness, ahead of most of his colleagues, that while the war lasted the need was to work through government to secure worker objectives. The scheme was also more than a broad concept; it was closely argued and bore the imprint of one who understood from first-hand experience the mechanics of what he was advocating. GM chairman Alfred P. Sloan contended that automobile plants were unsuitable for defence production, but in a letter to the *New York Times* Reuther answered technical criticisms of the Plan's feasibility, arguing persuasively that at the Cadillac plant in Detroit precision parts for the Allison aero engine were already being manufactured, using machinery that duplicated existing automobile plant equipment.[4]

However, the idea of unions having an equal voice with management in industrial policy-making was too much for the business community, and the Plan as originally conceived was rejected by the employer-dominated Office of Production Management. In the aftermath of Pearl Harbour, parts of the scheme were eventually adopted in a diluted form. A cutback in passenger car production was decreed, yet auto firms still delayed over conversion measures for many months, while large numbers of workers who might have been engaged in defence production remained unemployed. Reuther continued to campaign for a role for organised labour in the conversion process, on one occasion in March 1942 debating the issue with General Motors' chairman Charles E. Wilson on the radio programme 'Town Hall Meeting of the Air'. It was Reuther's contention that, with trade union participation, the process could have been completed rapidly, whereas in the event it dragged on well into 1942.

The plan for aircraft production was not the only one that Reuther was to issue during the war. With Eddie Levinson's help, he proposed a scheme under which the big three automobile companies would combine their efforts to make a standard model military tank; before the end of the war, he was also floating plans for reconversion and post-war production. James Wechsler wrote that Levinson had been responsible for creating a Reuther legend. But far from Reuther being an invention of Levinson, an alternative view is that it was Reuther who had the imagination to seek out this top newspaper man and woo him into the UAW. That Levinson was attracted by the idea of working with Reuther, who had yet to reach the highest office in the union, was a measure of the latter's magnetism.[5]

In 1942 Reuther was appointed to membership of the National Advisory Board of the War Production Board and the War Manpower Commission's Labor–Management Policy Committee. In these roles he worked closely with Sidney Hillman who, from the outset, had been the labour movement's senior figure in the Office of Production Management. With the creation within that body of a Labor Production Division in 1942, Roosevelt was evidently of the view that Walter Reuther would be an appropriate person to head it, but his name was not put forward by the labour movement. However, he now moved in high circles and counted people such as Under Secretary of War, Robert Patterson, and Solid Fuels Administrator, Harold Ickes, as his friends. A significant product of his campaigning on defence matters in government circles was that he began to have access to the White House through an acquaintance with the President's wife, Eleanor Roosevelt. Reuther had been introduced to her in 1941 by the liberal James Loeb, and shortly afterwards visited her at Hyde Park. There were to be many more such visits in the years ahead and theirs was to blossom into a close friendship. Whenever he found difficulty in obtaining a hearing in the administration for his ideas, Reuther would go to see Mrs Roosevelt.

Ironically, at the very time that Reuther's talents were coming to the notice of the administration, the Federal Bureau of Investigation (FBI) under J. Edgar Hoover began to compile a voluminous file on him as a subversive. Hoover was convinced that, throughout his life, Reuther was a communist, and he tried hard to alert the White House of the danger of appointing him to administration agencies. A proposal to assign him to the Department of Labor's innocuous Safety Device Board prompted the ever-suspicious Hoover to warn the President's Secretary in May 1940 that while in Russia Reuther had studied 'Agitation propaganda'. In the midst of the *500 Planes a Day* campaign, Hoover wrote to the Attorney General informing him that Reuther had been educated at Lenin University, Moscow and had been trained in street fighting. The FBI file was constantly updated, with details amended to include each new batch of gossip and rumour. Much of the material seems to have come from an agent who was a former employee of the Fisher Body Company, a UAW member who was part of the Addes (i.e. communist-leaning) faction of the union. An internal FBI memo to Hoover in September 1941 indicates that Reuther had been considered a candidate for custodial detention.[6] The author of the memo, John Bugas, was to become the Ford Motor Company's top labour relations manager in the 1950s. No action was taken by the White House on Hoover's warnings in these years, but the FBI file would grow and provide a routine source of ammunition to be leaked and used against Reuther by his business and political enemies in years to come.

Of course, Reuther was far from being a communist, and anti-Stalinism was now a significant element in his political philosophy. In the constant jockeying for the succession to the leadership of the UAW, he was always ready to draw attention to the fact that George Addes, the secretary-treasurer and, on occasion, Frankensteen and R. J. Thomas, followed the party line or at least allowed the communists to do their thinking for them. 'Red-baiting' was a charge that would often be made against Walter Reuther, and at times the spectre of communism was invoked when, in reality, his own position did not differ greatly from that of his rivals. Nevertheless, he understood very well the essentially conspiratorial nature of party activity in the labour movement, and the fact that 'red-baiting' was itself a slogan to ward off internal criticism of the communists' frequent arbitrary changes of line.

After a lull lasting a couple of years, the internal factionalism of the UAW flared up again in 1941 when the Reuther supporters at the union convention succeeded in passing a resolution, against the protests of Addes and Thomas, barring communists and fascists from holding union office. Behind the move lay resentment over the ultra-militancy of communist-led sections of the union in some major strikes before the entry of the USSR into the war on the side of the Allies in June 1941. However, Reuther's zeal in tackling the communists rebounded against him and he struggled to secure re-election to the executive board. He was considerably embarrassed by having recently been deferred from military service on the grounds that he was his wife's sole support: May Reuther was in fact his secretary. CIO and UAW leaders had intervened with the Draft Board to retain him in his key post with the General Motors Council of the Union and he was actually appearing at a federal mediation hearing regarding a threatened strike at GM on the day he was due to present himself before the Draft Board. The result was that he became the subject of taunts from his opponents, who referred to the Reuthers as 'the Royal Family', who would rather face cameras than bullets.

A year later the union's convention was a more tranquil affair, the opposing groups burying their disagreements now that America was in the war, and with contemporary rhetoric proclaiming the aim of 'victory through equality of sacrifice'. In 1942 Reuther seconded Addes's nomination for secretary-treasurer and Addes reciprocated by seconding Reuther's successful bid for election to one of the two newly created posts of vice-president. A quiet transformation of industrial relations was now being brought about; collective bargaining was becoming a routine practice and subject to greater bureaucratisation as part of a trade-off for union participation in a multiplicity of government regulatory bodies. Under the rubric of equality of sacrifice, there was meant to be an end to wartime profiteering, a limit of $25,000 on all incomes, rigid price controls and rationing. Negotiated wages were limited by the War Labor Board's so-called 'little steel formula', originally devised to cover the 'little' steel corporations such as Republic and Bethlehem Steel, under which wartime increases were restricted to 15 per cent, regardless of the cost of living (it actually rose 45 per cent during the war). Militancy was discouraged (strikes were forsworn) and union leaders found themselves largely engaged in presenting briefs to the War Labor Board. Earlier than most people, Reuther had understood that the traditional union role in collective bargaining would be restricted and that the need was for labour to exert its influence through wartime administrative agencies. Without such an approach, it is difficult to see what role the unions would have been allowed to play. Nevertheless, some of his fellow UAW officers complained that in frequent dealings with government in Washington he was indulging in what were essentially extracurricular activities.

Reuther's hope was to turn these special circumstances of wartime to advantage and to influence the government in the direction of progressive reforms. On the advice of his brother Victor, the CIO's Washington office hired a gifted economist, Donald Montgomery, to head a department emphasising consumer needs. Working with Montgomery, Walter Reuther was delegated to represent the UAW before a variety of consumer agencies. This association was to have a major impact on Reuther's approach to trade union issues in years ahead. But although in 1940 he had been among the first to see the possible benefits to be gained in working through government channels, by 1943 it was beginning to be clear that labour representatives were being relegated to advisory roles in administration agencies. Reuther now recognised, before many others, the importance of retaining labour's defensive armoury as evidence grew that the sacrifices of wartime were not being evenly shared. Wage restraint was effective, but the other elements of Roosevelt's equality of sacrifice programme were honoured more in the breach than in the observance. With ever-increasing support for repressive labour legislation, it was also evident that Congress's fight against trade unions was almost as fierce as its fight against Hitler.

The willingness or otherwise of the union to defend its members' interests became the focus in 1943 of a bitter debate in the UAW over the virtues of piecework. Communist supporters in the union had already unsuccessfully proposed the surrender of premium payments for overtime work. Now, however, an even more determined campaign was waged by the party nationally to have trade unions accept pieceworking arrangements which the UAW had previously rejected on the grounds that they invited the possibility of speed-up of work. Reuther refused to accept wage incentive schemes at General Motors, with the result that the Communist Party attacked him in the press. In the *Detroit News*, party leader Earl Browder wrote: 'Labor will be unable to give leadership until it settles accounts decisively with Lewis, Reuther and Co.'[7] At the convention in Buffalo later in the year, debate on this once again divided Reuther from Addes and his followers, the latter arguing for a more flexible policy that would have opened the door to piecework. The outcome was that the delegates supported Reuther decisively; Addes came close to being defeated as secretary-treasurer, while Reuther was elected ahead of Frankensteen as first vice-president. In the same year, Reuther resigned from his advisory position with the War Manpower Commission, sensing a growing tide of militancy among the membership and wanting to distance himself from administration labour policies, which were increasingly unpopular.

The same convention saw Reuther and Addes bitterly divided over rival policies for racial equality in circumstances where racial tension had assumed deadly serious proportions in Detroit. Thousands of southern blacks were moving to the city in search of jobs, discriminatory employment practices were prevalent, and housing conditions in the black districts of the city were deplorable. Strikes by white auto-workers had taken place in protest at black demands for an end to discrimination. And a three-day race riot in June 1943 had left 34 dead. Both Walter Reuther and George Addes now supported the appointment of a Director of Minorities in the UAW, but they disagreed over whether or not this should involve a guaranteed seat on the executive board for a black representative. On grounds of formal democracy, Reuther was strongly against positive discrimination, or 'Jim Crow in reverse': black and white members had to have identical rights. Yet his position was also influenced by a belief that communists were supporting positive discrimination in a cynical attempt to cultivate electoral support from the black section of the membership. The clash was indicative of the way in which the issue of communism was dragged into almost every debate within the organisation. Trade union issues could not be treated simply as such: matters of principle were approached by both camps in terms of how they might help or hinder their aspirations for leadership, and an essential difference between the rival camps was whether or not they could count on the support of the communists.

Feelings of relative deprivation and a sense that the burden of war was not being evenly shared fed a mood of shop-floor resentment that built up throughout 1943 and 1944. The UAW, along with other unions, was committed to a no-strike pledge, but a growing number of unauthorised strikes took place as workers followed the militant example of John L. Lewis's Mineworkers' Union, whose aggressive tactics in disregarding the no-strike commitment had clearly paid off. In the auto industry the union leaders found themselves presiding over a situation in which they were losing control. And yet the logic of persisting with the no-strike pledge was strong. In wartime conditions, every strike led to allegations from the business community and the press that labour was sabotaging the war effort. Congress was increasingly disposed to legislate against trade unions, and the CIO leadership believed that to revoke the no-strike pledge would be to commit organisational suicide.

In 1944 a rank-and-file caucus independent of the Reuther and Addes camps emerged in the UAW, arguing the case for immediate abrogation of the pledge. At the union's Grand Rapids convention that year, some 36 per cent of the delegates supported the new grouping.

Reuther had already distanced himself from those in the leadership who were willing to disarm completely in the interests of the war effort. Now he attempted to steer a delicate course between the rank-and-file caucus and Addes, who supported retention of the no-strike pledge. His proposal was to distinguish between civilian and military work and to abandon the pledge in the former case, while retaining it in firms that manufactured munitions. However, it was too clever a manoeuvre to appeal to the delegates and was derisively shouted down. The rank-and-file caucus were not strong enough to carry their own proposal, but nor would they go along with the proposals of Reuther or Addes. The issue was left to be resolved by referendum ballot which resulted in the maintenance of the status quo. The whole episode had been damaging for Reuther. He had lost badly; many of his own supporters had deserted him, and he was well beaten by Frankensteen in the barometer vote for first vice-president.

This was a salutary experience, and during the next twelve months Reuther worked hard to restore his credibility among the rank and file, all the while identifying with the growing shop-floor militancy. His calculation was that most of those drawn to the rank-and-file caucus were his natural allies who would return to his camp in the fullness of time. Early in 1945 he called for union representatives to withdraw from the War Labor Board unless the little steel formula was abandoned. On the executive board he voted against the disciplining of wildcat strikers. By the summer of 1945 he was arguing in favour of the taking of a strike vote to back up the union's demand for a large pay increase, and he was calling for a new referendum on whether to adhere further to the no-strike pledge.

The end of the war was in sight and difficult questions now presented themselves regarding the basis on which labour would seek to restore its position in peacetime while catching up on ground lost in the war. Reuther was gearing up to offer a militant lead, but his approach was not to be simple wage militancy. An indication of Walter Reuther's thinking in the latter part of the war is contained in a memorandum prepared in September 1943 by his brother and close colleague, Victor, who held the post of assistant director of the UAW's War Policy Division. It set out a philosophical approach for American labour which prefigured much that would become Reuther policy in the years ahead.

The memorandum began by criticising both Lewis's ultra-militancy, which was intensifying public antagonism towards labour, and the communist line, under which labour subordinated its interests to the war effort without adequate assurances of protection. As against these two positions, Victor proposed a third course in which labour would forge a radical popular alliance with other groups. There was, he argued, a need to break down the barriers of prejudice which isolated labour from farmers, technicians, professionals and other middle-class workers. This had to begin with a 'theoretical revision of outworn concepts of labor's ideological role in the struggle for economic democracy'. The history of the rise of fascism, he maintained, had demonstrated the inability of labour alone to combat reaction. At the same time he challenged the orthodox left interpretation of the Russian Revolution and its relevance for understanding the dynamic of developed capitalist countries. Here the numerical strength of the middle classes was increasing; they held the balance of power and tended to identify with the ruling elements in society. 'The extent of anti-labor sentiment in America today, when the issue of basic social change is not yet clearly defined,' Victor Reuther wrote, 'gives evidence of the inclination of the middle classes to resist labor's social advance.'

The logic of this pointed to the need for a progressive coalition of forces as the first order of business for the labour movement. It was necessary to convince labour's potential allies that the unions were determined to advance the welfare of the community as a whole. Unions needed to demonstrate sincerity of purpose and morality of motives by means of an accelerated and enlarged programme of public relations. It would require unions to undertake internal reforms to lend strength to their claims to democratic self-government, responsibility and concern with the public welfare. Racketeering and collaboration with employers, to the detriment of community welfare, had to be stopped. Meanwhile, joint action with other social and civic groups around community projects and public activities such as civil defence, education, social services, housing, public health, race relations and war relief, needed to be emphasised on a much broader scale, while playing down the 'endless clamor' for wage increases and closed shops.

In reviewing Roosevelt's wartime record, which had led to growing suspicion of him in sections of the labour movement and worker apathy in the 1942 congressional elections, Victor still calculated that the President would receive the backing of the trade unions if he chose to run again in 1944. In that case he argued for a change in their relationship:

> In supporting President Roosevelt . . . labor must break down the pater-
> nalistic psychology which has given rise to a labor attitude that attributes
> to him an exaggerated degree of progressivism and power. Support for the
> President must be predicated on a program of social action, and not on
> personal loyalty to a great man. While, for the time being, he is the ablest
> democrat available for labor to work with effectively on a national scale,
> he is powerless to act decisively in behalf of the progressive cause without
> strong backing from the unions and other progressive elements.

What this pointed to politically was the need to build a new grouping through which to press for a realignment of the Democratic coalition. The new progressive grouping that Victor Reuther envisaged labour building would be free from the reactionary influence of southern feudal Democrats. 'The rise of a labor party, or third movement, must be timed to coincide with the realization by farmers, white collar workers, professionals, etc., that they cannot longer entrust their destinies to either the Democratic or Republican parties.'

In programmatic terms, the younger Reuther called for labour to start thinking immediately about the possible pattern of a demo-cratically-planned post-war economy, combining the practical features of consumer co-operation, social ownership, expanding free enter-prise unrestricted by monopoly controls, and government ownership of public utilities and banks. Such union policies would lay the ground-work for a post-war society 'embodying the spirit of community en-deavour and co-operation, without either completely smothering individual initiative or plunging into a bureaucratic statism or collec-tivism'. Practically, it would necessitate government guaranteeing social security for all, eliminating monopoly controls, cultivating the growth of consumer and producer co-operatives in competition with non-monopolistic free enterprise, and encouraging the development of democracy in industry with a minimum of state intervention 'by stimulating labor participation in management through free contrac-tual relationships between unions and employers'.[8]

Walter Reuther's 1944–5 proposals for post-war reconversion through a Peace Production Board incorporated much of the spirit of his brother's memorandum. In March 1944, in a radio broadcast, he talked of the post-war need to fight a war against poverty and human insecurity, using the same determination as had been used in the battle against fascism. In the *New York Times*, he argued that advances in technology during the war had made it possible to create wealth in three-quarters of the time that it had taken before the war, and he debated the implications of this for work patterns with the shipbuilding tycoon, Henry Kaiser, and President of the Chamber of Commerce, Eric Johnson. With Brendan Sexton, UAW leader in the Willow Run bomber plant, he compiled a plan, *Are War Plants Expendable?*, in which the two proposed that the Ypsilanti plant be used to turn out modern railroad cars and prefabricated houses for social need.[9] In May 1945 Reuther submitted to a special meeting of the CIO executive board a 'Wages and prices programme for conversion' which focused on a number of linked issues: the implications of increased labour productivity for price restraint, a guaranteed annual wage, and effective rationing and controls.[10] In addition, an economic brief that he prepared jointly with Donald Montgomery and submitted to the Office of Price Administration at the end of June 1946, argued at length the case for wage increases without any compensating price increases. It was the first time that an American union in collective bargaining had made such a conscious attempt to win the consumer as an ally.

Reuther's concept of wages based on ability to pay took on particular relevance when on 16 August President Harry S. Truman issued Executive Order 9599 permitting wage increases provided that they did not cause price increases. The stage was now set for Reuther to lead the post-war bargaining round, demonstrate his militancy and parade his novel social thinking. On 18 August, he submitted the UAW claim to GM – a 30 per cent wage increase without consequent price increases. Similar demands were served at Ford and Chrysler.

The negotiations began in October and, as part of his strategy, Reuther asked for the sessions to be opened to the press, but this was refused. He therefore arranged for a stenographer to attend the sessions and presented the press with his own account each night. Throughout the negotiations little serious bargaining took place: the GM spokesmen paid little attention to the presentation of the union case, claimed that Reuther's argument was basically socialist, and pointedly refused to accept the central plank that ability to pay was relevant to a discussion of wages. To help win the propaganda battle,

Reuther invited a prominent group of church, education and civic leaders to come to examine the transcript of the negotiations and issue their findings. This National Citizen's Committee, under the chairmanship of Dr Henry Hitt Crane, issued a ten-point report supporting the union position. The device of calling on the services of a panel of distinguished people to pass judgement on union bargaining positions was one that Reuther would make considerable use of in the future. His understanding of the weapon of publicity was second to none, and in the course of these negotiations, union locals were kept supplied by the well-oiled Reuther machine with extensive documentation for use in seeking favourable publicity in their own community.

On 7 November 1945 GM offered 10 per cent, which the union promptly rejected. Reuther now played his second major card, offering to arbitrate the dispute if GM would open its books and demonstrate its inability to pay the increase demanded. GM refused the offer and the strike began. It was now that other CIO leaders began to have misgivings about the Reuther strategy. Most major unions had negotiations pending, and there was a reluctance to follow Reuther in insisting on wage increases without price increases. Philip Murray and Reuther met in Pittsburgh in December and had a sharp disagreement over his bargaining approach. Murray had no intention of following the line in the steel industry negotiations that he would soon be leading, and at his request, the UAW leaders responsible for the Ford and Chrysler negotiations now abandoned the strategy.

Reuther's approach was intriguing: it clearly put the union on the side of the consumers, while the call to 'open the books' seemed to pose a central challenge to GM as a capitalist concern. There were a number of editorials in the *New York Times* attacking the strategy as a threat to private enterprise. Reuther countered:

> The grim fact is that if free enterprise in America is to survive, it has got to work: it must demonstrate more than an ability to create earnings for investment; it must master the technique for providing full employment at a high standard of living, rising year by year to keep pace with the annual increase in technological efficiency ... The fight of General Motors workers is a fight to secure *truly* free enterprise from death at the hands of its self-appointed champions.[11]

On a practical level, the approach raised a number of important questions. How would the ability-to-pay argument apply when the demand was for industry-wide bargaining? What would happen in companies such as Ford which were financially troubled? What would be its relevance in a depression when profitability was reduced? The answers offered did not convince everyone, and sceptics drew the conclusion that the Reuther approach was not intended for serious application, but was merely an eye-catching publicity stunt. His strategy had far-reaching social and economic implications, yet, as critics pointed out, he did not develop them. It was a halfway stand – implicitly rejecting the kind of unionism which acquiesces in the capitalist status quo, while not yet ready to state that rejection openly. As Howe and Widick note, it was an excellent illustration of Walter Reuther's own social views, with all their difficulties and internal contradictions.[12]

A fact-finding body was appointed by President Truman to examine the case. GM now improved its offer to 13.5 cents, but then walked out of the hearings after learning that ability to pay would be a relevant consideration. The Board's recommendation of a 19.5 cents increase, with no compensating price increase, was duly rejected by the company, although it was still little more than half the union's claim. Meanwhile the strikers found themselves increasingly isolated. A strike by Murray's steel workers had begun, but was settled after four weeks when Truman reversed his earlier policy and announced that price increases would be allowed to compensate for wage increases. At Ford and Chrysler, the UAW had also settled for 18–18.5 cents without making an issue of ability to pay. And finally the ground was cut from underneath Reuther when on 9 February 1946 the United Electrical Workers (UE) at GM settled for what was by then the going rate of 18.5 cents without informing Reuther of their intentions. He regarded this very much as a stab in the back. Given that the UE was communist-led, the episode was bound to fuel the bitterness between the Reuther camp and the communists. Without a strike fund, and the members at GM suffering great hardship, the UAW called off the action on 12 March after 113 days. Though some minor concessions were gained to make the final settlement more palatable, the UAW was forced to accept the 18.5 cents that had long been on offer, and automobile price increases were not long in following. Reuther felt betrayed by his fellow union leaders and did not attend the full final session of the negotiations.

A whispering campaign against Reuther's leadership of the negotiations was now set in train as, with the benefit of hindsight, colleagues dissociated themselves from the strike strategy. People who had been party to the early strategic decision-making now began to claim that the venture had been mistaken. The arguments were variously that Reuther was wrong to tackle GM in isolation – all three main car manufacturers should have been targeted for strike action; that the UAW had broken ranks with the CIO in not following the strategy of the parent organisation, and that the action had commenced too early and before industry was back to full peacetime working. Union president R. J. Thomas complained that the strike had begun too early and had gone on three weeks too long. Yet he had been a member of the executive board which approved the bargaining strategy, and on this Reuther supporters did not constitute a majority. The 'one at a time' approach which the communists (among others) now criticised was not a Reuther innovation, but merely a continuation of UAW practice since 1937. Whether or not there was in fact a CIO strategy for the bargaining round is not at all clear – Murray appeared not to be convinced that strike action was inevitable. Much of the criticism was clearly opportunistic, as in the communist *Daily Worker*, where early support for challenging the concept that the employer was the sole judge of whether or not his business could pay a living wage gave way to criticism as the policy implications of a change in party leadership were felt.

The UAW convention at Atlantic City was less than two weeks away, and Reuther made it clear that he would challenge R. J. Thomas for the presidency of the union. His decision to run for the leadership was not taken suddenly: it had been under review in the Reuther caucus since the previous summer. The militant tactics deployed at GM had been an integral part of the effort to establish his leadership credentials in the eyes of the membership. According to Addes, during the negotiations with GM Reuther had discussed with him on several occasions the future leadership, proposing that there should be a three-way contest for the presidency between himself, Addes and Thomas. If Addes won, he should support Reuther for the secretary-treasurership and vice versa. But Addes would not agree to this deal and remained loyal to Thomas.

Although the GM strike had not been a success, it was still possible for Reuther to present himself to the membership as the only contender with the drive and the imagination to lead the union through what was clearly going to be a very uncertain period. With a flair for self-publicity, he was the union's best known figure. A *Life* feature on him in November 1945 commented that 'his growing fame rests less on his achievements as a union leader than on his talent for offering solutions to national problems and getting them well-publicized'. [13] His rivals, practitioners of 'penny ante unionism', signally lacked his bold approach to the issue of reconversion, and against the recent background of conservative leadership in wartime when the patriotism of Thomas, Addes and their communist supporters had gone hand-in-hand with a fair measure of strike-breaking, it was not difficult for Reuther to present himself as the most militant candidate. The press tended to report Reuther's challenge as a manifestation of anti-communism, while Thomas and Addes represented the contest in terms of personalities. In fact, Reuther's campaign emphasised practical issues of union policy, advocating a programme to end the animosity bred of factionalism and calling on delegates to think about 'political consciousness' rather than 'power politics'. Despite the fact that Philip Murray effectively gave his endorsement to Thomas, Reuther convinced a majority of the large number of uncommitted delegates that he was best equipped for the job. He was was elected president, albeit with a wafer-thin majority, but the delegates also elected an executive board that was overwhelmingly anti-Reuther in composition. After the ballot, R. J. Thomas refused to shake hands with him: the omens were not good for internal union harmony.

The war years were important for Reuther, allowing him to derive valuable experience of Washington politics. The tripartite structures within which labour operated were a model whose re-establishment in peacetime he would never cease to advocate. His prominent position in the War Manpower Commission and the War Production Planning Board, and the opportunity that it afforded him to publicise his ideas for labour's role in war and peace, helped to establish him as a national figure. The war years were also an extended period of manoeuvring for the succession to the leadership of the UAW. Here he and his rivals, Addes and Frankensteen, were all vigorously engaged. Reuther had been among the first to recognise that the ground rules for the conduct of industrial relations would have to change during wartime, and he rapidly moved into the mainstream of political debate. However, he was also quicker than the others to sense in 1943 a growing mood of discontent on the part of the union membership over the uneven burden of wartime hardships, and the issue of piecework and the no-strike clause became important matters of dispute among these rivals.

Although Reuther's fortunes slumped in 1944, the positions he adopted generally on trade union questions appealed more to the members, and he made skilful use of his rivals' identification with the ultra-patriotic Communist Party as he set about burnishing his own militant credentials. In 1945 he had two decisive advantages: as executive board member responsible for General Motors negotiations, he was perfectly positioned to stamp his personal leadership on the first post-war round of negotiations in mass production; and by this time he had also developed an attractive philosophy of community trade unionism for peacetime that emphasised the role of the worker as consumer as well as producer. His bargaining demand for a wage increase without price increases and his challenge to GM to 'open the books' were viewed by the corporation as a frontal assault on the rights of management and were answered in kind, and when his fellow UAW officers withdrew their support for his strategy, the way was open for him to challenge for the presidency as the more militant candidate. Up to this point the UAW membership were inclined to be wary of Reuther's driving ambition. But now he seemed to offer the best programme for the future, and the members duly gave him their cautious support.

4 The new man of power

Walter Reuther's presidential victory in March 1946 marked the start of the most intense period of factionalism in UAW history. With but a third of the members of the new executive board supporting him, and with his three fellow officers – secretary-treasurer Addes, and vice-presidents Leonard and Thomas – openly hostile, Reuther had the title to leadership but little of the substance. In the eighteen months until the next convention, a furious battle was fought by the two sides for absolute control of the organisation. In the course of this, Reuther's supporters were a coalition of predominantly young, militant members, often drawing their inspiration from socialist-leaning figures, and the well-organised Association of Catholic Trade Unionists (ACTU), who shared both Reuther's opposition to communism and his moral approach to trade unionism and labour–management relations. On the other side, the Addes–Thomas–Leonard group was now more cohesive than ever and operating in much closer collaboration with a Communist Party in the process of abandoning its wartime quiescence and advertising its claim to militancy.

The Addes faction was incensed that Reuther had secured the presidency and were determined, if possible, to neutralise him in that position. A document apparently drafted by Maurice Sugar, the fellow-travelling legal counsel of the UAW, which circulated within the Addes group stated that they must use their majority on the executive board immediately to prevent the new president from completely 'capturing' the union. They must make no concessions on staff appointments, and there would have to be a head-on clash with a definite victory for the majority if Reuther moved to dismiss any of the leading staff members associated with Addes. There were to be no deals: 'Reuther is not on an equal bargaining plane with the Board. In fact, as matters stand right now, he has no bargaining power at all . . . The Board must . . . assume complete control over the appointment and disposition of the personnel in the administration of the International

Union.' [1] A tight discipline was enforced within the Addes faction, and on any issue involving a challenge to Reuther, all were expected to support the group line.

Addes fired the opening shot within weeks of the 1946 convention. Without consulting the president, he issued a statement, originally drafted by the Communist Party, for adoption by the UAW executive board which repudiated Reuther's 'ability to pay' theory of wages, advocated industry-wide bargaining, and also opposed 'Catholic, Protestant, Negro, Jew and Red Baiting'. The executive board was claiming the right to make policy independent of the president. Reuther would later complain that he had been forced to eat humble pie from the date of his election. [2]

Battles between the two sides were fought over control of union finances and the staff appointments that might provide one or other with a tactical advantage. The General Motors strike had left union funds seriously depleted, dues-paying membership had fallen considerably from its wartime peak, and at an early stage Reuther was forced to borrow $250,000 from Hillman's Clothing Workers and Murray's Steelworkers to pay the wage bill. In straitened circumstances, staff reductions were necessary: competitive empire-building had produced a bloated staff of 500. Reuther proposed that cuts should be made where organisational needs dictated, rather than with a view to reducing the strength of the rival faction. But this approach was blocked: [3] Addes would not agree to jobs being 'taken out of politics', and Reuther would make political capital out of this record of waste and partisanship when, a year later, he stood for re-election.

At national level, a patched-up compromise allowed Addes to appoint the director of research, and Thomas to claim for himself control of the Competitive Shops Department, responsible for the numerous small supplier firms in auto. Meanwhile, Walter was able appoint his brother Victor to be the director of education and another faithful colleague from Socialist Party days to the directorship of the Publicity Department and editor of the union newspaper. These two appointments were critically important for Reuther in the faction fight, giving him a channel of communication to the membership at large and control of the programme through which a new generation of local leaders would be schooled in the art of union politics. In the event the main thrust of the education and training provided to thousands of members in weekend and summer schools was to equip Reuther supporters with the political and organisational skills to fight the immediate battle. As long as he had these resources, the hostile executive board could not rein him in completely. The positive use he made of these two departments would be manifest at the next convention.

Accepting that there was blame on both sides for the friction, Reuther made an attempt to promote internal harmony, calling for more give and take. He told the executive board in December 1946 of his idea for a conference of selected groups representing different strands within the union to thrash out their problems and do away with factionalism. Yet it was indicative of the climate in the union that this failed when his opponents leaked to the press his confidential proposals before any progress could be made. Over many months there were rancorous exchanges within the executive board over the inadequacy of the minutes that were kept of their meetings, with Reuther calling for verbatim records. There were challenges over the ruling that communists should not hold office. The Addes faction censured Victor Reuther's Education Department for issuing what was seen as political rather than educational literature. Reuther tried to dismiss from his post Irving Richter, a UAW lobbyist in Washington and a key member of the Addes faction, whom Reuther was convinced was a secret communist, but the executive board blocked this attempt. At one point during his first term of office, the president had to threaten to refuse to sign pay cheques in order to secure concessions from his opponents.

CIO President Murray described the UAW faction-fighting as a state of 'complete moral degeneracy', aiming his criticism mostly at the Addes people. Although Reuther had begun his presidency without Murray's support, as 1946 progressed the two found themselves increasingly in the same camp. The CIO president was becoming more and more concerned by the influence that the communists were seeking to wield in the organisation, and he backed a resolution condemning this at the 1946 CIO convention. Because of Reuther's opposition, the part played by communists in his union had long been a matter of contention. With the coming of the Cold War, the issue of communism in trade unions became a subject of general debate in labour's ranks. As Bert Cochran comments, 'the Red issue in the midst of the Cold War was a time bomb'.[4]

The boldest attempt to freeze Reuther out of basic policy-making, and the most open challenge to his leadership by the Addes faction, came in summer 1947 with an attempt to negotiate a merger between the UAW and the communist-led Farm Equipment (FE) union. Although an amalgamation of these two organisations with overlapping constituencies made sense, this rushed initiative was clearly conceived as a way of boosting the voting power of the Addes group within the UAW. Reuther was excluded from the negotiations with FE, and the decision to recommend the terms of merger to the membership was taken without proper notice. The terms included provisions for FE to preserve their autonomy in policy matters, to retain their bloated full-time staff (a bonus for the communist faction), and to safeguard their craft principle of organisation, and for the UAW to take over FE's dubious finances. Reuther opposed the whole project and he finessed the manoeuvre by urging rejection in his president's report, which he circulated to all members without notifying the executive board. The proposal was duly rejected in a referendum ballot, giving the Reuther cause a welcome fillip on the eve of the October 1947 convention.

Reuther went into the Atlantic City convention confident of being able to defeat his opponents. Only two weeks earlier at the CIO convention, Murray had come out firmly against the communists, and with Addes clearly tied to their camp, the tide was set to run in Reuther's favour. Before the convention he flew to Pittsburgh to tell Murray that he intended to run a full slate of candidates with a view to sweeping Addes from office and warned the CIO President not to intervene. Thanks to the educational work of brother Victor during the previous year, the Reuther caucus was highly organised and effective. Caucus meetings were rumbustious affairs held in the Chelsea Hotel where one observer recalled a husky character acting as doorman shouting: 'This way way to the Reuther caucus; that way to chaos.'[5]

Reuther was very much in the ascendant. Despite the handicap of his minority status over the previous eighteen months, he had shone above his fellow officers. Addes was personally popular and his views were shared by many members who had no communist sympathies. But neither he nor the other officers had a policy programme as plausible as Reuther's. Moreover, they had not enhanced their own standing as a result of their negative campaigning and their identification with a scurrilous piece of anti-Reuther literature circulated on the eve of the convention entitled 'The Boss's Boy' which sought to portray him as the preferred candidate of big business. They accused him of supporting the speed-up of work and piece-work wages, which gave him a splendid opportunity to remind delegates just who had been the real evangelist of such measures during the war. His opponents also circulated a story that he was likely to be the vice-presidential running mate of conservative Senator Robert Taft in the 1948 presidential election and that he supported Taft's anti-labour legislation passed in the summer of 1947, the Taft–Hartley Act.

The major policy debate at the convention was over Taft–Hartley, which aimed at shifting the balance of power in labour relations decisively in favour of the employers, restricting the political activities of trade unions, while seeking also to drive a wedge between communism and the labour movement. Passage of the Act has since been seen as a climacteric in American labour relations, and attempts have been made to portray it as an issue that separated right from left in the UAW, with Reuther firmly on the right. The reality is rather more complicated. The pressing issue facing the convention was whether or not the union should comply with the provisions of the Act which required elected officers to swear affidavits that they were not members of the Communist Party. The entire leadership of the UAW were agreed that such a requirement was both a breach of civil liberties and discriminatory since no comparable requirement was placed on employers. The practical question was whether they should refuse to sign – in which case they lost the protection of the labour relations legislation and left themselves open to membership-raiding by other unions – or whether they should swear the affidavits under protest and seek to challenge the constitutionality of the Act while still ignoring its limitations on political activity. Reuther's intention was to follow the line of the CIO, but the Congress gave its affiliates no clear lead on how they should act. Other unions were breaking ranks and agreeing to comply with the legislation, and in these circumstances a poll of the UAW executive board before the convention revealed a majority in favour of signing the affidavits. Reuther sided with the majority whose position was upheld by a large majority of convention delegates. However, in standing with the majority on this question, Reuther was branded by his opponents as a supporter of Taft–Hartley which, they said, should be renamed the Taft–Hartley–Reuther Act.

With a dominant personality, Reuther stood out from his rivals. To some he could appear impetuous and excessively ambitious; but the majority who supported him did so because of the appeal of his ideas. He talked persuasively about 'our new kind of labor movement'.[6] He told the convention: 'We are building a labor movement, not to patch up the

old world so you starve less often and less severely; we are building the
kind of labor movement that will remake the world where the working
people will get the benefit of their labor.'[7] Besides his consumerist
philosophy of collective bargaining, his policy programme included
support for an economic bill of rights and progressive legislation for a
minimum wage; expanded social security; a national health programme; redistributive taxation; low-cost housing, and the creation of
a national daily labour newspaper. He denounced factionalism, not least
because of the damage it did to the union in collective bargaining, where
employers were able to divide and rule locals. He was consistent in his
opposition to Stalinism, but he avoided the crude, conservative anti-
communism that was to characterise American society during the Cold
War. When the Governor of Michigan accused Addes and his associates
of being communist captives before the House Un-American Activities
Committee in March 1947, Reuther condemned the reactionaries of
the country for waging a red hunt whose ultimate victims would be not
communists, but all effective labour leaders. 'We must fight against . . .
home-grown varieties of fascists', his report to the 1947 convention
declared, ' . . . and we must guard against their technique of smearing
every decent liberal and progressive with the brush of communism. On
the other hand we must fight against the Communist Party and their
efforts to employ the same smear technique in reverse by branding as a
Fascist and Red-baiter everyone who has the courage to oppose or to
criticise the Communist Party line.'[8]

Reuther was elected by a huge majority – 5,539 votes against fewer
than 350 shared by his two opponents – and carried a full slate of officers
with him. Addes, Thomas and Leonard were all defeated and quit the
union. On the executive board the overwhelming majority of members
were now Reuther supporters. He dismissed several prominent officials, including legal counsel Maurice Sugar, research director James
Wishart and lobbyist Irving Richter, along with seventy-seven union
organisers. Reuther justified shedding the latter in terms of the need for
economies. Critics argued that he was engaged in a wholesale purge of
opponents, but in truth his action fell short of that. It was normal for
staff closely identified with defeated candidates to lose their jobs: but
Reuther prevailed on some newly-elected executive board members to
restrain them from a house-clean of all their regional staff, and on
balance he retained more people who had opposed him than he fired.[9]
With comprehensive control of the organisation for the first time, he

called for 'teamwork in the leadership and solidarity in the ranks'. This was to be the new watchword, replacing the old slogan of 'local autonomy'. It reflected the fact that the union leadership would now be more centralised – and factionalism was out.

In the years ahead, Reuther used the power of appointment to build up his support within the union. Cynics have often claimed that factionalism in the UAW had been, at bottom, nothing more than a scramble for union jobs, and no doubt there was always an element of that present. Some have gone further and argued that there was no significant policy difference between Reuther and Addes, and that the one thing that divided them – Reuther's anti-communism – amounted to less than a programme.[10] A more accurate way of stating the position is to say that Reuther's was essentially a programme of social democratic reform. Despite their rhetoric, what the Communist Party stood for was no more radical, and they supplied Addes with much of his thinking. But where the two camps differed crucially was that the democratic credentials of the Reutherites seeking to promote these polices were rather more convincing than those of the communists. With regard to communist supporters in the UAW, Reuther's policy now was not to repress them by administrative means (though the union had barred them from office since 1941 and would continue to do so), but to flush them into the light of informed opinion and defeat them by argument.

Some argue that in giving Reuther such a clear mandate for his programme, the delegates unwittingly destroyed the basis of the finely balanced system of internal union democracy that had existed since the departure of Homer Martin in 1939. With R. J. Thomas as president initially holding the balance between the Reuther and Addes groups, the two sides had had to compete for membership support, and competition, so the argument ran, did not detract from the effectiveness of the union.[11] Reuther disagreed: factionalism had damaged the UAW's ability to perform, often leaving a vacuum where national policy should have been and allowing local unions to decide on their own uncoordinated activities. In any event, by the late 1940s many UAW members were weary of internal fighting and believed that democracy could be maintained without it. Under Reuther's undisputed leadership, there was a greater spirit of co-operation and less political manoeuvring. Significantly, at the first post-convention meeting of the executive board, held in Detroit, Reuther invited all the members to his home for Thanksgiving dinner, something that would have been unthinkable under the previous regime. In caucus meetings he now felt able to concentrate on discovering the flaws in the union programme rather than mobilising his supporters to defeat the rival group.

However, the caucus was not without its own internal differences. Some members were relatively conservative, while others, such as the new secretary-treasurer Emil Mazey, were more radical than the president. In the late 1940s a socialist commentator, Irving Howe, sensed that the conservatives in the group had become dominant, benefiting from the prevailing atmosphere in American social life, while the more radical Reuther supporters had not been very coherent or self-confident.[12] Yet others judged that under Walter Reuther the UAW became the most profoundly class-conscious and community-conscious union in the United States.[13]

The concentration on the worker-as-consumer was reflected in the big co-operative programme that was started in Detroit where six warehouses, a gas station and a general store were opened to serve workers belonging to some twenty local unions. As education director, Victor Reuther developed a highly professional programme, using radio and television as well as the press to transmit the union's message to members. The UAW purchased a Detroit radio station, WDET-FM, in 1949 which they proceeded to operate as a public welfare station, reaching an audience estimated at 50,000. Unfortunately, FM sets became too expensive for workers to buy – the union was ahead of its time in this regard – and the station was sold in 1952. Still they continued to produce radio and television programmes for broadcast on other outlets, including a fifteen-minute summary of the news each night, a Sunday evening TV programme, 'Meet the UAW–CIO', and a popular radio programme entitled 'Shift Break', timed to coincide with workers driving to the plant.

It was in the field of collective bargaining that UAW conservatism was said to be on the rise, and the evidence that some people pointed to was was the growth in bureaucratic control of the bargaining process. To evaluate the debate about this, it is helpful to have some sense of the evolution of collective bargaining in the auto industry in the 1940s.

After the first breakthroughs in 1937, little progress had been made in collective negotiations. The internal conflicts of the Martin period contributed to a large number of sectional strikes that were disruptive of solidarity and were often unpopular among the membership. But as the union was reconstructed following Martin's defeat, the first attempts to impose more centralised control of labour–management relations was made. The leadership required union locals to adhere strictly to grievance procedures, and the executive board called on them to use other workers as temporary replacements for small groups who tried to shut down plants in wildcat action. A more disciplined form of militancy began to emerge. Between January and November 1939 there were only two unauthorised strikes, while the number of officially-led actions increased.

In 1940 GM agreed to recognise shop stewards, the absence of which had been a factor in shop-floor conflict since it meant that there was no approved union spokesman in a position to settle disputes. In the same year the UAW made a breakthrough in the method of handling grievances with the agreement to appoint a permanent umpire who would arbitrate such cases. GM had been unwilling to cede such influence to a third party, and over the coming years the union would attempt to widen the umpire's powers while management resisted the pressure. Meanwhile, the company insisted that work standard disputes should not be covered by this mechanism and the UAW retained the right to strike over them. At Ford, the company was not finally forced to concede union recognition and bargaining rights until 1941. In accepting the new regime, the company was transformed almost overnight from being the most anti-union employer to the one offering the most liberal terms. It agreed to a union security clause and the automatic deduction of union dues – the 'check-off' – (Henry Ford was intrigued by the prospect of being the union's banker!). There was no reference in the first Ford collective agreement to production standards, and in any case the existence of a vigorous shop steward system, a product of the long battle for a union presence in the firm, enabled workers to disregard many managerial controls.

Thus, in the major companies there were elements of increasing bureaucratisation and routinisation of bargaining procedures, side by side with informal practices based on rank-and-file autonomy and self-confidence. Since the days of unquestioned employer dominance, autoworkers had wanted formal protection against arbitrary management, notably through the establishment of grievance procedures and acceptance of the principle of seniority, both of which were inclined to spawn bureaucracy. At the same time rank and file union members had come to recognise the benefit of being able to respond flexibly and spontaneously on the shop floor when the situation required it. Between these two positions there was an inevitable tension that would never be fully resolved. What degree of centralisation was necessary for the achievement of wider union goals? How much did members stand to lose through centrally – imposed restrictions of their freedom to engage in local industrial action?

Under the watchful eye of the War Labor Board (WLB), the war years saw significant increases in the bureaucratic controls over bargaining procedures. The arbitration of grievances grew in the context of the no-strike pledge; wage increases were regulated by the little steel formula, and payroll deduction of union dues and 'maintenance of membership' – a half way house to a union shop – were encouraged by the WLB as a compensation for wage restraint. In general the union position in non-economic matters was enhanced in wartime: management's freedom to deploy and discipline labour was curtailed. The price that unions paid was to forfeit influence in economic matters, and this was the cause of the growing militancy in 1943 and 1944 which provided the background to the 1945–6 strike at GM.

In the early post-war years other factors also increased the tendency for union members to lose some of their local autonomy and for the gap between membership and leadership to widen. In 1946 Ford set about re-establishing its managerial rights over work standards and discipline and sought to make the union responsible for policing its own delinquent members. In return for matching the GM wage increase, the company insisted on the right to discharge workers supporting wildcat strikes and to discipline people failing to meet production standards. At the same time shop stewards were replaced by a much smaller number of full-time 'committee men' responsible for processing grievances in a more bureaucratic fashion. Similarly, at Chrysler the union agreed to cease processing grievances for workers guilty of leading wildcat strikes, while the umpire's powers in such matters were reduced. In general the employers were intent to claw back rights eroded during the war. In this they were assisted by new technology which eliminated worker-paced production and undermined the power of shop-floor groups. There was also a growing tendency for umpires to evolve the notion of 'negative leadership' under which local leaders were held responsible for strike action even if they had played no role in sparking the breach of contract. The pressure was on them to become contract policemen.[14]

The early development of bureaucracy in labour–management relations was not something for which Reuther bore major responsibility. He had negotiated the introduction of the umpire at GM, but he had also been responsible for securing the recognition of shop stewards. The wartime routinisation of bargaining that the WLB presided over affected all industries, not just automobile production. And until he had become president with undisputed control, bargaining at Ford and Chrysler was outside his purview. Here the employers' successes in restoring the right to manage and in bureaucratising the shop steward function had been wrested, not from Reuther, but from his rivals in Addes's circle. Communist supporters themselves, who would later be his biggest critics on this issue, did little to oppose the conservative routinisation of collective bargaining. Opponents represented Reuther as one who had bowed down before the provisions of the Taft–Hartley Act, a measure designed to ensnare labour–management relations in a web of legal restrictions. Yet he was far from being alone in this respect, and without a shift in the political balance in the country, it is hard to see what else he could have done that would have been effective.

However, Reuther's consumer/community-oriented approach to bargaining was a strategy that presaged more centralisation in negotiations. He was never willing to be satisfied with short-term, parochial wage bargaining since he was playing for altogether bigger stakes. For him, union decisions in collective bargaining had to be understood in the context of the mix of macro-economic pressures that influenced profits, prices, investment and the level of employment. And 'unity in the leadership: solidarity in the ranks' implied that bargaining goals would be pursued in a more systematic, disciplined fashion than had previously been the case.

Not until 1948 did the results of collective bargaining begin to reflect the Reuther philosophy. In that year the agreement at GM linked wages and prices through a then novel cost-of-living escalator clause, with a further link between wages and national productivity trends established through the introduction of the 'annual improvement factor' under which wages were to be increased automatically each year in respect of productivity growth. Although GM President Charles Wilson was credited with these innovations, he was almost certainly responding to Reuther's concern to establish a link between wages, prices and productivity, even if, as Reuther's successor Leonard Woodcock believed, Wilson had hopes of devising a bargaining-proof mechanism that would leave little left for the union to negotiate over in the field of wages. Wilson's formula owed even more than that to UAW pressure. It represented an about-face for the company which, only weeks before, had been hoping to negotiate a system of incentive wages until it saw, in a parallel set of negotiations at Chrysler that involved a bruising seventeen-day strike, just how militant the UAW was still prepared to be. On the other hand, the 1948 agreement with GM represented the first move away from one-year to two-year contracts. In years to come they would be even longer, and critics saw this as part of the process under which conditions of work became less susceptible to rank-and-file influence.

Although the 1948 round of collective bargaining bore Reuther's imprint, he himself was absent from the negotiations, the victim of an assassination attempt. Returning home from the office on the evening of 20 April, he was shot through his kitchen window by an assailant with a shotgun and received serious wounds to his arm and ribs. He almost lost the use of his arm, and was absent from work for many months. As with the assault on him at his home a decade before, his attacker was never brought to justice. Such evidence as was collected by Senator Kefauver's Crime Committee and by a private investigator hired by the UAW suggests that Reuther had fallen foul of the Detroit underworld, possibly linked to a disaffected communist opponent of his in the UAW — his one-time friend, Melvin Bishop. Before the shooting, Reuther was aware that a Sicilian gang, led by Santo Perrone, had been acting as a strike-breaking agency for companies such as Briggs in return for the award of lucrative scrap metal contracts. Reuther's call for the investigation of this operation is likely to have made him a target for Perrone. But Perrone was also associated with Melvin Bishop, a former UAW director in Detroit's East Side whom Reuther had dismissed in 1947. Reuther believed that officers of the Detroit police may also have been involved in the assassination attempt and certainly made no serious effort to solve the crime: hence the UAW's engagement of a private investigator. The FBI also refused to conduct an investigation, even though they were already maintaining close surveillance of Reuther and despite being urged to intervene by the Attorney General's office. J. Edgar Hoover's position in this matter was clear: 'Edgar says no,' was the Bureau response to calls for action. 'He says he's not going to send the FBI in every time some nigger woman gets raped.'[15]

The scandal of FBI neglect was underlined just thirteen months later when Victor Reuther was also shot through the window of his Detroit home, losing the sight of one eye. Again, police attempts to trace the assailant were amateurish. Only after an attempt was made to blow up the UAW headquarters when Reuther was present in the building, just before Christmas 1949, did the FBI open an investigation. Yet no-one was ever brought to trial, and the body of the UAW's private investigator was later fished out of nearby Lake St Clair. The immediate effect of these attempts to silence the Reuthers was that Walter was forced to live the rest of his life under conditions of tight security in a secluded house, accompanied always by a bodyguard and provided with a UAW-issue bullet-proof car.

Once Walter Reuther was back at work in 1949, what would become a distinctive feature of his approach to collective bargaining was his emphasis on negotiating fringe benefits that increased the economic protection available to workers. One of his first major bargaining achievements of this kind was to agree a non-contributory pension scheme for Ford workers in 1949 – the first negotiated scheme in mass production industry – under which retirement income for the average worker was tripled. 'Too old to work, too young to die' was the slogan Reuther coined in leading this campaign. Not only was it a breakthrough in establishing a negotiated pension scheme, but the result was a *funded* pension scheme and, as such, something that many employers were reluctant to concede because of their fear of unions having some control of major investment power.

However, critics pointed to the fact that this new interest in negotiating fringe benefits, an approach that inevitably involved national union leaders and professionals more than rank-and-file representatives, blossomed at the same time that the union was acquiescing in the neutralisation of the shop steward's function. It was in this respect that Reuther found himself open to the charge of fostering bureaucratic collective bargaining. Some claimed that members themselves were less interested in fringe benefits than in securing basic protection against the speed-up of production that followed hard on the heels of management's attempts to reimpose control of the shop floor. In practice, this was how Reuther opponents presented the options in the late 1940s, and for some time the focus of the battle between the two styles of unionism was at Ford.

The late 1940s saw the production of the first new model cars since

1941. With them came new production standards that led employees to claim frequently that work was being speeded up. It was now a buyer's market, auto manufacturers were competing with each other to lower costs, and workers were paying the price in greater effort. Reuther recognised the problem: there was a concerted drive by the employers to increase the pace of work, and members had to be protected by the union. He argued that this task needed to be undertaken at a high level rather than through wildcat action, and bargaining procedures had to be fully explored first. Part of his answer was to cut down the length of time it took the union to process grievances.[16] This led his critics to claim that he was thereby collaborating with management. In fact, 386 strikes were authorised by the UAW in the twelve months to April 1949, and some 200,000 workers went on strike in the first four months of 1949 alone.

However, at Ford the question of speed-up became a political football between pro-Reuther members, who controlled the local union, and Reuther opponents, who urged the need for spontaneous action on the grounds that he had effectively sold out on the issue. Complicating the picture was the fact that negotiations over the pension scheme were about to start, and management appeared to be attempting, through the deliberate speeding-up of work, to provoke the union into premature strike action. Yet Reuther was equally anxious not to allow the UAW to be diverted from its primary target: 'on the one hand we stand uncompromizingly in opposition to any efforts on the part of corporations, large or small, to exploit their workers and get lower unit costs of production out of further exploitation of the human equation in production,' he told the executive board.

> On the other hand, we are not going to be provoked nor maneuvered into irresponsible, irrational wildcat action on the part of the local unions . . . We also ought to realise that in this period, nothing ought to get us on a detour, when every effort and every bit of energy of this union ought to be keeping our main drive down the broad highway in terms of our 1949 economic demands . . . which are coming up in Ford very shortly.[17]

In May 1949 a strike lasting three weeks was authorised at the River Rouge plant over the speed of work, less than a month before the contract was due to be renegotiated. Yet for Reuther it was a distraction from the main issue and so he reached a compromise with management under which an arbitration panel would rule on whether temporary increases in the speed of production were detrimental to health and safety. It was a fudge and it helped earn the president a reputation for shirking the real challenge to labour over increases in the pace of work. Union policy was that these had to be negotiated and were strikeable issues: in practice they were often a *fait accompli* with no action threatened or taken.

Reuther has sometimes been accused of taking the easy option in focusing on fringe benefits as a bargaining objective. The implication is that such concessions were relatively easily won from prosperous corporations, whereas a battle over management's right to control the intensity of the production process would have been fought tooth and nail by employers.[18] However, that is to minimise the scale of the union's achievement in providing members with new economic protections, and it also ignores the unfavourable political context which dictated that decent health and social security benefits be won in the field of collective bargaining or not at all.

By the late 1940s labour's earlier hopes that the government would introduce a comprehensive range of welfare state benefits had died. Labour would have to seek the equivalent through negotiation with employers. But Reuther also recognised that it might be possible to use such negotiations as a lever with which to raise the value of the basic state benefits that already existed. Therefore, in negotiating the pension plan with Ford, the union deliberately defined its demand for a $100 per month pension in terms of the combined value of company and state benefit. In practice, it meant that the employer now had a strong incentive to lobby government for an increase in state pension benefit in order to minimise his own contribution to the total, and this is exactly what transpired. With major employers suddenly converted to the cause of higher state pensions, 1950 saw the first basic improvement in the Social Security Act since its enactment fifteen years earlier.

Though Reuther was much more inclined than the average business union leader to see the need for political activity to secure what collective bargaining was unable to achieve, he nonetheless had great faith in collective bargaining as a potential weapon for general social advance. With unemployment mounting during the 1949 recession, he was due to discuss the problem with President Truman, but before doing so he told his executive board that ultimately the solution would be found in collective bargaining through its contribution to bringing about a fairer distribution of wealth. As compared with bargaining, all the federal job-creation schemes such as housing and river valley developments were, he argued, only stop-gap measures.[19] In years to come, critics would note that the failure of the labour movement to win sufficient gains for the greater community weakened the prospects for a political alliance between labour and non-labour groups.[20] However, to what extent the trade unions were masters of their own destiny in this matter can be judged only by examining the political context.

The wartime Roosevelt administration, dominated as it was by businessmen, lost much of its attraction for organised labour, and towards the end of the war there were growing calls for the creation of a third party. Walter Reuther had not supported a move in Michigan to launch a labour party – the Michigan Cooperative Commonwealth – in 1943–4. Immediately following Roosevelt's victory in 1944, his brother Roy wrote to him urging the case for CIO endorsement of an independent political movement of trade unions to operate on a permanent basis, not just six weeks before every presidential election.[21] In late 1945 Victor Reuther also wrote that the time was ripe for labour to divorce itself from the two old parties and to start to build a new national party. Throughout 1946 the CIO became more and more disillusioned with Truman as hopes for the creation of a welfare state began to fade. Walter was careful not to commit himself on the idea of a third party. Yet one thing he was convinced of was that the Socialist Party was too dogmatic to fill the bill: such an organisation would need to grow organically from the American soil. In practice this meant positioning himself somewhere to the left of the Democratic Party.

In the summer of 1946 Victor Reuther supported the calling of a conference of all progressive groups in the belief that both established parties were incapable of solving the country's problems.[22] However, when the conference met, hopes of it leading to the creation of a mass labour party were dampened by Philip Murray's strictures against Communist Party interference in the affairs of the trade unions. A political third force would have to be as independent of the Communist Party as it was of the Democrats or Republicans. As it happened, some felt this was not really the time to be talking about independent labour action at all. In the non-presidential election year of 1946, an extremely conservative Congress was returned, while in Michigan the Republicans elected 95 out of 100 state representatives and even won a majority of the vote in labour's stronghold of Wayne County. Reuther was sensitive to the deteriorating political climate in 1946. In the course of a radio broadcast in May of that year he had vigorously defended CIO calls for government intervention in the economy, against the scare campaign being run by the business community that this would lead to a 'government-controlled economy'. However, after the depressing election returns of November his tone was necessarily more conciliatory and he spoke now of unions and management joining together to solve problems. 'I'd rather negotiate with General Motors than with the government,' he asserted, 'General Motors has no army.'[23]

Within two months of the congressional elections the groups that had attended the Conference of Progressives were split into two factions: the Progressive Citizens of America (PCA) which, under the guidance of the Communist Party, went on to form the Progressive Party and launch Henry Wallace's bid for the presidency; and Americans for Democratic Action (ADA) in which Walter Reuther became a leading light. ADA appealed to Reuther because, while independent of the Democrats, it retained the possibility that it might succeed in pushing the party into adopting more progressive policies, particularly if it put down roots among the labour movement and avoided being merely a gathering of well-intentioned liberals. At the founding conference, he expressed the belief that liberals among the Democrats were inclined to be gadflies who lacked a serious approach to politics:

> ADA must not be a refuge for tired exiles, a home for aged and indigent slogans. ADA must be a tool to sharpen and use. We need more dash, more boldness . . . we didn't build our [UAW] union on virtue alone. We had to tangle with spies and thugs and get our heads cracked . . . I'm trying to suggest the kind of hardening of the will we need as we go down the road . . . ADA, to me, is the beginning of a militant, aggressive political movement. That or nothing, in my opinion. If it is to grow . . . it must lose a certain provincialism I detect in it at present . . . ADA must go to the grass roots. It must go into the steel towns and the auto towns . . . The accent . . . must be on the rank and file. Generals are no good without an army. If ADA gets too top-heavy, it will fall on its face . . . If we are to build the creative alternative to totalitarianism of the right and left, then, I believe, we have no choice but to regard ADA not as the left wing or tail of any established party, but as the matrix from which a new movement shall arise. Our watchword must not be: back to the New Deal, but forward from the New Deal.[24]

Reuther had come to regard Truman as 'hopelessly inadequate',[25] and with other ADA leaders he cast around for a replacement for the presidential nomination. His own preference was for liberal Supreme Court Justice William O. Douglas and he was responsible for the judge appearing as a guest speaker at the CIO convention in November 1947. However, Truman was not to be dislodged and Reuther was forced to live with him as candidate in 1948. The central issue for labour in that election was the fact that the anti-labour Taft–Hartley legislation was on the statute books, and that only a Democratic victory offered the prospect of repeal, while Wallace's candidacy could at best split the labour vote. Reuther distanced himself from Truman, and urged his members to concentrate their efforts on congressional and gubernatorial elections rather than the presidential one. Meanwhile the union looked beyond the election, calling in March 1948 for a genuine progressive political party.[26] In August 1948 Reuther wrote that he did not propose to spend the rest of his life just running from one fire to another, trying to put out with a leaky bucket a blaze that should never have started in the first place. He now made a pledge that political action would have the first call on his time as president.[27]

Truman's unexpected victory upset the plans for an independent party. Wallace received only 2.2 per cent of the Michigan vote and a derisory 3.5 per cent of the vote in Wayne County. With justification, he regarded Reuther as the greatest single obstacle to his party. Democratic Party success was largely a victory for trade union organisation and effort. There was a feeling that the prospects for labour within the Democratic fold had now radically changed. As the socialist Max Lerner put it, they had moved from a New Deal party inspired by a great leader to a New Deal party which has taken over its own leadership.[28] Reuther was due to attend a UAW education conference the day before the presidential inauguration in 1949 where he had been expected to announce steps for a new party, but the strategy now altered. 'The thing we are determined to do,' he told the *New York Times* correspondent, 'is to avoid any narrow, premature, sectarian approach. We must make a real try to influence the old parties. If we find we cannot, then the move for a third party must come from the bottom and have a very broad base. It must not be a palace revolution like the abortive Wallace candidacy.'[29]

An added reason for Reuther having second thoughts about the Democrats was that since 1947 in Michigan the state CIO had de-

veloped a unique alliance with reform-minded members of the party,
and UAW members were urged to become active in its affairs. As a
consequence, the liberal Mennen Williams had been elected Governor, bringing to an end a long period of Republican dominance in
Michigan politics. As the leading influence in Michigan CIO affairs,
Reuther now developed a particularly fruitful political relationship
with Williams over the next decade. The lesson seemed to be that the
Democrats could be seen as America's labour party, and at this
juncture Reuther effectively turned away for good from the idea
of independent political activity. Third-party proposals were
advanced from time to time at UAW conventions in the 1950s, but
Reuther deflected them while insisting on the UAW's independence
of party ties: 'Nobody owns us,' he would say, 'we don't belong to anybody and we won't be the tail of any political party
kite.'[30]

It was a crucial turning point and many would say it sealed the
political fate of American labour. The UAW policy adopted at the
union's next convention was to try to build an independent machine
within the Democratic Party. Reuther's preference for this course is
perhaps understandable, given that in 1949 his close friend and former
socialist George Edwards was defeated in the Detroit mayoral election, the fifth time that Detroiters had rejected the chance of electing a
labour mayor. If this was the pattern in such a relative trade union
stronghold, what hope was there for independent labour representation generally?

The communist-inspired Progressive Party campaign of 1948 was
but one element in a mix of Cold War developments at work on the
international and domestic scene whose effect was to cause a deep
fissure within the CIO. Anti-communist hysteria was building up in
America and the UAW was just one of several CIO unions in which
internal faction fights fed off, and in turn contributed to, this
phenomenon. However, it was in the UAW that the outcome was
most decisive. Riding high as leader of the CIO's largest affiliate,
Reuther not only led the opposition to the Progressive Party but also
spearheaded the move to commit the Congress to support for Marshall
Aid, which many in the labour movement believed had the potential to
become a true 'people's programme'. 'The Marshall Plan has not been
blueprinted,' he told the 1947 CIO convention.

I think you and I, the people of America, ought to fight like hell to blueprint the Marshall Plan. The Marshall Plan is an idea; it is a good idea . . . the people of Europe are being told: 'Do you want Joe Stalin or do you want Standard Oil?' I say they want neither . . . give us our place around the councils in Washington just as they did during the war so that we can make this a really and truly people's movement . . .[31]

At the following year's convention, in the immediate aftermath of the Democratic victory in 1948 and fresh from convalescence, he pressed for more decisive measures to be taken against those unions that had supported Wallace, that were still politicking over Taft–Hartley (which Truman had promised to repeal), and that continued to oppose the Marshall Plan. It was, he said, time for them to 'get clear in the CIO or clear out of the CIO'.

However, it would take another twelve months of Reuther's pressure before Philip Murray steeled himself to take firm action against the dissident organisations. Severe measures were called for by the UAW president: 'The body politic has a bad case of cancer, and we have either got to save the cancer or the body,' he told the 1949 convention. 'We have come here to cut out the cancer and save the body of the CIO.'[32] The gathering duly proceded to amend the CIO constitution so as to permit investigation of communist-dominated unions who were held to be working in the interests of the USSR. As a result, eleven affiliated unions, accounting for over 20 per cent of CIO members, were expelled. These were draconian measures, the long-term effect of which was to blunt internal debate within the CIO and signal its demise as a crusading organisation. From now on, it would seek social change by means of partnership with government and industry, not through labour insurgency.

Some held Reuther primarily responsible for these developments which cost the labour movement dear. However, labour politics in the late 1940s were more complicated than that, and the fact is that the Cold War largely eliminated the option for genuine radical politics. As an individual Reuther was in no position to resist contemporary political pressures which were to lead to the isolation of the left; nor could he escape the political and economic logic of an era in which the mentality of business unionism grew with the realisation that America was entering a period of unexpected economic prosperity.[33]

From the intense factionalism of 1946–7, Reuther emerged as the unquestioned leader of the UAW. There were several reasons for this. His ideas had more appeal to the rank and file; the positions he took on trade union issues made better sense to them; his style of leadership conveyed a freshness and openness, and as a shrewd tactician he simply outmanoeuvred his opponents. By 1947 the tide was also flowing strongly his way, not least because of the growth of anti-communism in the country on which he was able to capitalise. Opponents would claim that he overplayed the anti-communist card and that the CIO suffered badly as a consequence. The UAW that emerged in this period was more centralised and cohesive than before. While for some the demise of oppositional groups and the cut-and-thrust of internal politics caused a loss of vitality, for others the transformation meant that the UAW was at last able to concentrate on serving the interests of the members. In fact, it remained a very dynamic organisation with a social and community orientation that many found highly attractive.

In negotiations, Reuther began to reveal the shape of things to come with a more concerted approach to corporate-level bargaining over wages and fringe benefits, while demonstrating a reluctance to give the ranks their head in shop-floor struggles over production questions. Critics argue that collective bargaining under Reuther became more bureaucratic. This process certainly gathered pace in the 1940s, but the trend preceded Reuther's presidency and drew added impetus from Taft–Hartley, though there are those who question whether his opposition to the legislation was quite as strong as it might have been. In fact, he followed UAW policy which was to comply with the Act while challenging its constitutionality and working politically for its repeal. This was, arguably, a sounder approach than that followed by some of his opponents, which was to support Wallace in 1948 and risk the return of a Republican administration committed to keeping the legislation. Politically the late forties were a difficult period for the labour movement: a strong conservative mood was sweeping the country, and it is hard to see what the unions could do but ride out the storm. Reuther's decision to steer clear of the idea of a third party oriented to labour was understandable in the circumstances, but the consequence was to cement the link between the trade unions and the Democratic Party, and in the long run that was to prove an alliance of doubtful value.

Reuther was, then, one of a generation of radicals who came to regard leftist politics as a dead end, but he never discarded his socialist background, and there were always a number of people around him who provided links to what remained of the American socialist movement and contributed intellectual yeast to UAW policy. If he was neither 'The American Radical' nor another Samuel Gompers, he was, as Bert Cochran has argued, a leader who blended together the practicalities of business unionism with a vision of reforming idealism.[34]

5 Union president in a conservative decade

Organised labour in 1950s America reflected two overriding influences – the Cold War and growing economic prosperity. It was a decade in which mature collective bargaining with a legalistic base and elaborate procedures, conducted by trade union professionals, yielded significant economic gains to workers and contributed mightily to stable and predictable industrial relations. Politically it was a decade of deep conservatism and retreat from the values of the New Deal and the early post-war optimism of labour radicals. Fratricidal strife in the CIO in the late 1940s had reduced that organisation's strength and blunted its cutting edge. The Cold War abroad, of which the CIO's travails were a by-product, and McCarthyism at home shifted the balance of politics such that for trade unionists to challenge the conservative consensus was to invite questions regarding their patriotism. Wider societal changes were also having their influence, and in the context of growing affluence and worker home-ownership, there was a tendency for what was known as the 'tuxedo unionism' of well-heeled labour bureaucrats to displace what remained of the proletarian thrust of 1930s insurgency.

Some see Reuther as a contributing architect of this settlement. He certainly set out to make the best of what was on offer, working within the system rather than challenging it head-on. The terrain of the 1950s was determined by external forces, and it was not open to one man or even one labour organisation to reverse the tide of world events. Like other labour leaders, Reuther had to stake out his position within it, and he did so by embracing the challenge of the new-style collective bargaining while attempting to enlist its services in advancing the frontiers of government social provision. Politically he came to terms with the fact that an independent party of labour was increasingly unlikely to succeed, while constantly seeking to build alliances with an array of progressive movements and organisations, and searching for a role for the UAW as a ginger group around the Democratic Party. He did not doubt that the American political system was capable of delivering the good life for his members: what was wrong was the programmes, the alliances and the will to act. In particular, he recognised that rigidities imposed by the Cold War acted as a sheet anchor in preventing social and economic change that would be to the advantage of working people. Uniquely within the labour movement, he devoted considerable energy to the forging of labour alliances abroad, whose effect, he hoped, would be to ease Cold War tensions and help generate an international consensus for democratic social reform.

With a secure majority on the UAW executive board, Reuther initially allowed his caucus to fall into abeyance. However, the absence of membership mobilisation on behalf of leadership policy proposals at the 1949 convention led to the defeat of the platform, and so the caucus was resurrected as an instrument of control. Under Reuther, the UAW boasted of its formal democratic structures, but in practice democracy tended to be carefully managed. Scope for rank-and-file influence declined in various ways: conventions were less frequent; the growth of a professional corps of full-time staff created a buffer between the ranks and the leadership, while elections were contested by rival lists of candidates for all offices rather than by competing individuals, making it harder for disaffected members to challenge the leadership. As president, Reuther controlled job patronage with the result that it was more difficult for executive board members to build their own power-base in rivalry to his. And his judicious use of the power of patronage helped him win over former opponents whose indebtedness to him now eliminated a possible rallying point for future opposition, while reinforcing the administration's liberal credentials.

Many, including some sympathetic to Reuther, maintained that he ran the UAW with the iron grip of an infallible man, his executive board reduced to a rubber stamp. It was the climate of anti-Stalinism that provided the immediate context for this development, but Reuther had long seen factionalism in the union as a debilitating influence, and in pursuit of organisational efficiency he was naturally drawn to a form of democratic centralism. This was the essential meaning of his slogan 'unity in the leadership, solidarity in the ranks', and welding the two components together was the Reuther caucus. Where previously this had been a broad-based group made up of hundreds of rank-and-file members, what counted now was the central caucus, comprising the members of the executive board, with its own rules and a mutual assistance pact. Caucus rules governing candidacies for election made it harder for members to challenge sitting officers and so reinforced the dominance of the leadership group. Prior to UAW conventions, a small rank-and-file caucus, chosen carefully by the executive board cabal, met to endorse candidates and policies being proposed by the latter. This procedure allowed an element of rank-and-file participation in what was otherwise a system of one-party government.

Rival caucuses that were formed from time to time were easily beaten back. Open opposition from communists was answered by constitutional changes which empowered the executive board to initiate action against disruptive party members of a local union rather than wait for local leaders to do so. The Ford members at the River Rouge plant provided Reuther's most serious opposition, and the local union was placed under administrative control of the national leadership in 1952 after its officers had abandoned a trial of alleged communists before the completion of proceedings. Two years before, a GM local had been put under trusteeship for claiming in its journal that the collective agreement signed that year was akin to the Soviet five-year plan. Local newspapers were brought under the supervision of headquarters and required to conform to the policies of the union. By such means, most organised anti-Reuther activity was rooted out in the early 1950s.

Carl Stellato, the president of the Ford local, became for a time the leader of the anti-Reuther forces in the union, but it was a very uneven contest. Stellato ran unsuccessfully for one of the posts of vice-president against a Reuther-supported candidate at the 1955 convention, but by that time one-party dominance of the union was all but complete, with fifteen of the eighteen executive board seats filled by acclamation. When Stellato was nominated to run against Reuther for the presidency in 1957, he quickly withdrew. In fact, no serious challenge to Reuther's own position was ever mounted after his defeat of R. J. Thomas. He was re-elected thirteen times, on the last occasion with 98 per cent of the votes.

However, it was not a repressive system of union government that Reuther ran. Unlike other American labour leaders, he did not seek to create an autocratic internal regime, and majority decisions were reached without strong-arm tactics. Without doubt, he really did try to involve members in the wider democratic process, and UAW-trained people were always prominent participants in community politics. Supporters maintained that he had a genuine concern for the need for a radical but responsible union opposition; that there were still occasional defeats for the leadership, and that he always allowed dissidents the chance to speak. He still believed that communism had to be defeated by exposure rather than by administrative means, and consequently its influence at the River Rouge plant was felt well into the 1950s. Political opponents were marginalised, but their civil liberties were defended: communists were barred from holding office, but the union went to law to prevent the deportation of a communist under investigation by the House Un-American Activities Committee. Reuther spoke of trade union office as 'a public trust, to be used for the advancement of the country's welfare'.¹ The ultimate protection of UAW members' rights was through a unique Public Review Board, established in 1957 against the background of allegations of widespread labour movement corruption. Accepting that union decisions had to stand the test of public scrutiny, the UAW appointed seven distinguished citizens to this independent board with full constitutional authority to review, modify, affirm or reject any decision made by the union with respect to individual rights.

From 1947 Reuther had been the second most powerful figure in the CIO after Philip Murray. When Murray died suddenly in 1952, Reuther was the obvious successor. Yet he was not the universal choice among CIO leaders: Steelworkers' president David McDonald disliked him, and that union's vice-president, Alan Haywood, was nominated to oppose him in what was seen as a calculated slight. Reuther won the election decisively, but in announcing the result to the convention delegates, Textile Union president Emile Reive wondered aloud whether the new president would have the necessary qualities of humility and understanding to make a good leader.

Humility was not Reuther's strongest suit, but in accepting the office he delivered a rousing speech, outlining his approach to the challenges facing the labour movement. There was a need to recapture the crusading spirit of the early days and to address the task of organising the unorganised. More than that, there was the job of educating and unionising the organised: transforming mere card-carrying members into people who had a sense of belonging to a great human crusade. It was necessary to find a way of raising collective bargaining above the level of a continuing struggle between competing economic pressure groups. The trade unions also had to go beyond collective bargaining and organise politically. '[Y]ou cannot raise the level of political morality in Washington,' he declared, 'until you first raise the level of political conscience on the part of the people back home.' The ultimate challenge was to tackle the wider problem of inequality in the world:

> There is a revolution going on . . . It is a revolution of hungry men to get the wrinkles out of their empty bellies . . . of people who have been exploited by imperialism and who are trying to throw off the shackles of imperialism and colonialism . . . The Communists didn't start it. They are riding its back . . . The Communists would have people trade freedom for bread and the reactionaries would have you believe that if you want to be free you have to be economically insecure . . . In the world that we are trying to help build, people can have both bread and freedom.[2]

However, the high-sounding idealism was now beyond the capacity of the CIO to deliver. There were continuing divisions among the affiliates and considerable tension between the leadership of the two largest unions, the UAW and the Steelworkers. Reuther recognised that the CIO was in failing health, and within days of being elected he met AFL president George Meany, and agreed to work for organisational unity. Negotiations between the two bodies proceeded over the next two years. Leading the smaller of the two sides, Reuther's idea was not to engage in a scramble for the top job, but to fight over issues of policy. His priorities in the merger talks included a purge of corrupt business unions; a racially integrated organisation; commitment to organising the unorganised, with the industrial unions of the old CIO having their own separately funded section, the Industrial Union Department (IUD); and an end to independent international activities conducted by the AFL's semi-autonomous Free Trade Union Committee (FTUC) which was led by Jay Lovestone, formerly the grey eminence behind Homer Martin.

The merger creating the AFL–CIO was consummated in December 1955. The AFL secured the two top posts, with Meany as president. Reuther became one of twenty-seven vice-presidents and head of the IUD, which claimed 7 million affiliated members and an income of $1.7 million. It was an apparently strong political base. Initial hopes were high for the merged organisation, but it was not long before tensions between the two wings began to appear. It later became clear that underlying this was a deep clash of philosophy between Meany and Reuther. The contrast between the business union leader and the social visionary was encapsulated in their remarks at the first UAW convention following the merger. Meany told the gathering: 'Trade unions are set up for a specific purpose and a very simple purpose – to advance the welfare and interests of the workers represented by the union, and when men are elected to office in a trade union, they are elected to office for that same purpose and no other purpose.' Reuther, on the other hand, insisted before the same body: 'It is the responsibility of the leadership of that movement to work together to build it more strongly, to make it more dedicated, and to make it more socially responsible in terms of its broad approaches to broad questions.'[3]

Issues of principle that Reuther thought had been agreed in the merger talks began to arise as points of conflict in the AFL–CIO, and the merged organisation proved in practice to be a conservative body bearing the clear stamp of the senior partner. The questions of recruitment, the position of blacks, racketeering and international policy all proved to be internal battlegrounds, though for the first few years Reuther's position was that, with good will, these problems could be ironed out through rational discussion. At the time of the merger, Reuther was a far better known figure than George Meany, and the expectation of the industrial-union wing was that the two would operate more or less as co-equal leaders. However, that was not how the Meany camp perceived the relationship, and in the years ahead it would become clear that Meany viewed Reuther as just one of the organisation's many vice-presidents.[4]

The most celebrated example of the growing maturity in collective bargaining was in 1950 when Reuther signed a five-year agreement with GM. This 'Treaty of Detroit', as it was called, renewed the annual improvement factor and cost-of-living provisions pioneered in the late 1940s. For the company, it was seen as a bold move that would guarantee industrial peace and allow GM to plan for the long term. For workers, it was to be a 'moving stairway to prosperity', though commentators also interpreted it as a sign that the union had come to terms with the requirements of capitalism and was accommodating itself to the authority of corporate management.[5] Of course, the issue was not whether the union was negotiating an accommodation with management – an eternal fact of life for trade unionism – but under what terms and with what protections. There was much speculation about the real significance of the agreement. GM encouraged the public view that the union had abandoned its concern to relate wages to profits and the wider interests of the consuming public, and that it had at last been forced to accept technological innovation. Reuther insisted that there was nothing new in UAW acceptance of technological change, but re-emphasised that technological progress must benefit the whole community.[6] There were union misgivings about entering into such a long-term agreement, but Reuther always believed that it could be reopened if necessary, and this proved to be the case in 1953. However, the experience of the five-year agreement was not one that the union cared to repeat, and in the years after 1955 a pattern emerged of collective agreements each lasting for three years.

Following the establishment of negotiated pensions and the twin formulae of the annual improvement factor and cost-of-living allowance as the basis for progressive wage increases, Reuther's next major bargaining objective was to secure a guaranteed annual wage for autoworkers. As a way of ironing out peaks and troughs in the employment cycle, the idea had its roots in the New Deal, when autoworkers argued that, if employers had to pay wages all year round, they would find a way of making employment more regular. Reuther began to focus on this target in 1950. The union aimed to impose a financial penalty on layoffs declared by the employers by means of benefits paid from a fund to which employers would be forced to contribute. An important emphasis of the union was to try to integrate negotiated benefits provided by the employer with state unemployment compensation in such a way as to give the major corporations a sizeable financial stake in the maintenance of full employment policies by government. There was also a counter-cyclical thrust to the proposal: the fund would soak up profits during times of expansion, while increasing the spending power of workers during times of recession. In Reuther's rhetoric, the guaranteed annual wage was 'more than a matter of economic justice to the wage earner; it is a matter of economic necessity to our nation, for freedom and unemployment cannot live together in democracy's house.'[7]

The long-term preparations that went into formulating the guaranteed annual wage demand were typical of Reuther's systematic approach, to bargaining. It took over two years to define the basic approach after which – and still two years away from collective bargaining – the full weight of the UAW's publicity machinery was brought to bear in putting the demand on the negotiating agenda. In this the UAW used its own radio and TV programmes, seeking to persuade the general public as well as its members of the logic of the demand. Reuther announced to his members in 1953 that the guaranteed annual wage would be the union's top priority in the negotiations of 1955. He talked about it as an inevitable development: it was not a question of *whether* they would secure it, only whether it would be won before or after a strike.[8] Likewise, he told the Michigan State Bar Association in November 1953 that he would not sign any agreement in 1955 without it containing a guaranteed annual wage. It was a typical Reuther bargaining tactic to induce fear into the other side by locking himself into a bargaining position at an early stage. Long before negotiations began, he gave management the impression that every union resource would be thrown behind the demand.[9]

To demonstrate that the union was acting responsibly and in the interests of the consumer, Reuther submitted the guaranteed annual wage proposal to the scrutiny of a Public Advisory Committee as had been done in previous rounds. Ten leading economists, including Alvin Hansen and Seymour Harris, were appointed to this body, and the scheme was revised in light of their criticisms. Meanwhile, employers launched their own well-funded campaign to discredit the proposal. The National Association of Manufacturers set out to raise $32m. to fight the guaranteed wage, and later they tried to make the proposal inoperable by securing court rulings that state and negotiated unemployment benefits could not be paid at the same time.

Against the threat of strike action, Reuther eventually secured agreement with Ford on what was termed Supplemental Unemployment Benefit (SUB). It was less than the guaranteed annual wage that he had originally envisaged, but the arrangement under which company and state benefit combined would pay workers 60–65 per cent of take home pay for thirty-four weeks when laid off was a significant breakthrough, representing an increase in unemployment benefit of up to 100 per cent in some states. It would take a series of incremental improvements over the next twelve years before SUB amounted to 95 per cent of straight time wages payable over a full year. Still, before the end of 1955, firms employing over a million workers had copied the Ford scheme, and in the next eight years more than double that number benefited from schemes that were modelled on the UAW plan. As in the case of state pensions, there was now an incentive for employers to press for higher government unemployment compensation since firms paid less in SUB in states where government benefit was higher. Largely as a result of this pressure, no fewer than thirty-three states increased the level of their compensation during 1955.[10]

These negotiations received world-wide publicity, and in June 1955 Reuther appeared on the cover of *Time*. Coinciding with the first shock waves felt in the labour market as a result of automation, it seemed to some that the UAW had secured the protection that meant automation could be faced without fear. Reuther himself did much to promote this line, and was prone to speak of it as a 'guaranteed wage' rather than as the more accurate Supplemental Unemployment Benefit. His critics have suggested that the guaranteed wage campaign was essentially a leadership initiative which failed to excite the rank and file.[11] However, it is arguable that the leadership had shown considerable foresight in negotiating at a time of buoyant employment a provision that would cost the employers little in the short run while certainly benefiting members in the medium and long-term. However, the victory at Ford did coincide with a wave of wildcat strikes called in frustration at the failure to resolve outstanding grievances on workplace issues. The bureaucratic grievance procedure was having difficulty in dealing with local problems, and for some the wildcat strikes were evidence that the gap between union and membership was ominously wide.

Reuther maintained his concern about the relationship between wages, prices and profits. Throughout the latter half of the 1950s and into the 1960s he continued to spar with the auto companies over their pricing policy and its relationship to inflation, a contest that necessarily spilled over from collective bargaining into the politics of national economic management. In 1955 exorbitant profits were being made by GM and Ford. Even after taxes they were still three times the average of all US manufacturing industry. Yet both companies announced price increases in 1955, using as an excuse the bargaining concessions they had recently made. The result was a sharp upward twist in the inflationary spiral, to which Reuther responded by calling for a congressional inquiry into pricing policy[12] while demanding that the big three reduce prices of 1958 models by $100. This proposal was to form part of the background to the 1958 collective bargaining round.

In 1959 Reuther proposed before a Senate Committee under Senator Estes Kefauver the need for legislation which would require advance notice and public justification of price increases by firms accounting for 20 per cent or more of the sales of any particular industry. It was not a call for price controls, but was intended to stimulate public awareness of the effects of corporate pricing policy. Because of the large profits being made, the union had demanded profit-sharing during the 1958 bargaining round. Reuther now reiterated the policy dating from 1946 that the UAW was prepared to confine its wage demands within the limits of whatever amount could be granted by an efficient firm operating under conditions of full employment without causing price increases.[13] The Kefauver Committee compiled damning evidence of price administration by GM. Competition had effectively ceased, and four GM executives effectively fixed prices for the entire industry. Prices and profits had far outstripped labour costs over a twenty-year period, and GM policy was to break even when producing at only 40 per cent of capacity. Yet in the Eisenhower years, 'an interregnum of largely ceremonial and absentee government' as Reuther termed it,[14] no legislation to restrain prices was likely. Reuther remained conscious that labour was failing to reverse the popular perception that unions were responsible for inflation. It was therefore necessary to mobilise liberal public opinion on the union side. And it was in this spirit that he had approached the 1958 round of collective bargaining.

The union demand was for an annual division of profits between shareholders, workers and the customers (in the form of reduced prices). Beyond a certain specified level of profit, corporate earnings would be distributed to shareholders, workers and consumers in the ratio 50 : 25 : 25. However, American industry was now in deep recession, one-third of the UAW's membership was unemployed, and with hardly any bargaining leverage Reuther presented the profit-sharing proposal in the mildest possible terms. It was a flexible programme, he claimed, tailored to fit the different economic situations of the larger corporations and the smaller companies. 'If the employer prospers, we expect a fair share, and if he faces hard times, we expect to cooperate . . . Our basic philosophy towards the employers . . . is that we have a great deal more in common than we have in conflict.'[15] Reuther told the British reporter of the *Sunday Times* that the profit-sharing idea was not a demand, so much as a mechanism: 'We're trying to find a rational means by which . . . [we] can attempt to work out in [our] relationship practical means by which you can equate the competing equities – in workers and stockholders and consumers.'[16]

To some extent, the pursuit of profit-sharing, which would be a goal of Reuther over the next decade, marked a change in direction for the UAW. Back in the late 1940s such schemes had been derided as employer gimmicks which passed on to workers the burden of fluctuating profitability, and encouraged them to break solidarity with union members elsewhere. Profit-sharing sought to make capitalists out of workers, and 'has a smell of money about it', explained a UAW Research Department document.[17] Yet the demand now presented was intended as a way of financing fringe benefits, rather than linking worker income to profits. Reuther believed strongly that this sort of arrangement would help to even out inflationary pressures, especially where there was little competition between firms. In such a situation, a profit-sharing plan would enable workers to share in the high profits in periods of peak demand, and would diminish the appetite for outsize wage increases in times of slack demand and low profits.

However, the demand was rejected and the negotiations with GM in particular were conducted in an atmosphere of mutual recrimination and name-calling. To defuse this, Reuther wrote in emollient terms to the president of GM that labour and management had a joint responsibility to the entire nation which transcended their responsibility to their own groups: 'Recognising . . . that as human beings we are imperfect and fallible, we should be willing to accept aid and guidance from others who, being less directly involved, can take a more objective view of our problems than can either the Company or the Union.' The smaller American Motors Corporation had already agreed to appoint a panel of ten church leaders selected by the company to give moral guidance, not to arbitrate, on the issue of profit-sharing, and Reuther told GM that he would accept the same panel fulfilling the same role in this situation.[18] Though he practised no religion, Walter Reuther always maintained positive contacts with the clergy through the Detroit Religious and Labor Fellowship, and his periodic appeals to men of God to act as mediators enabled him to claim the moral high ground in the eyes of the public even when, as on this occasion, the more materialistic men of industry remained unmoved.

Enjoying a bargaining advantage as a result of the high level of unemployment, GM calculated that Reuther would either be forced to agree to accept an extension of the 1955 agreement without further change, or blunder into a suicidal strike. Yet strike action was out of the question for the UAW. Its treasury was depleted as a consequence of a third of its members being laid off, and with GM attempting to squeeze the union's finances further by refusing to continue with the automatic deduction of dues, the UAW was forced to make major economies, laying off 100 field representatives and cutting pay by 10 per cent for staff remaining. Reuther was compelled to play for time throughout the summer of 1958, 'rocking and rolling', as he put it, and striving to hold the organisation together as management seized the opportunity to assert their authority in the plants. Eventually, the tooling-up period for the 1959 model season gave the union some leverage, and new agreements were negotiated with the major auto manufacturers that yielded modest gains, though not the union's major demands.

The 1958 negotiations again highlighted the fact that autoworkers were increasingly constrained by the formal bargaining and grievance procedures in their attempts to resist managerial pressure for more effort at the point of production. In these years of recession, the in-plant struggle was fierce, with management modifying the rights of union representatives, making grievance procedures stricter and pushing for higher work norms. At Chrysler, in particular, there had been a determined attempt by management to increase the pace of work in order to match productivity at GM. A major reorganisation of management personnel had taken place and long-standing work practices were under attack. There was also much rank-and-file resentment and frustration at the union since the leadership refused to sanction strike action until after the conclusion of the major contract negotiations.

Apathy and discontent grew in equal measure. Reflective of this was the fact that there had been vocal opposition to a proposed increase in union dues at the 1957 convention. Pensions, SUB and other fringe benefits were fine, but some members questioned their worth if they were financed by speed-up.[19] Reuther's caution in sanctioning any strike in the adverse conditions of 1958 was understandable, but the problem of how to respond to speed-up had existed for years and would continue throughout his leadership. Once the 1958 contract had been settled, the union agreed to allow local strikes on local issues in order to try to clear the backlog of unresolved grievances. This would become the pattern in future years, with major collective bargaining followed by a period in which industrial action could take place at plant level. But members tended to regard it as a poor substitute for the ability to strike speedily in defence of workplace conditions. Strikes over production standards were theoretically possible, but were only authorised very reluctantly by the union leadership. With firms able to transfer production from plant to plant, some local disputes could be won only by means of secondary industrial action, yet the UAW leadership were unwilling to defy Taft–Hartley on this issue. At the same time, rather than negotiate with local union representatives, plant management was often happier dealing with national union officers, who under Reuther's leadership had come to be seen as a force for 'responsibility'. A socialist autoworker critic of the Reuther regime blamed the union for having fostered an atmosphere of complacency in the ranks, promoting a blind faith in the union's powers. They were, he said, guilty of joining in the prevailing postwar ideology that held that basic social problems were being solved by American capitalism, and in this way the members were disarmed.[20]

By the late 1950s the number of authorised local strikes in the auto industry was on the increase as the leadership responded cautiously to rank-and-file discontents. With this went a subtle shift in the focus of collective bargaining from national to local issues. Significant breakthroughs in negotiations were harder to come by in the recession years of the late 1950s and early 1960s than previously, and one effect of the UAW's change of tack was to add to the leadership's difficulties in producing the dramatic contract settlements of before. Yet the shift in emphasis to the local level never amounted to a basic change in Reuther's bargaining approach.

In his presidential acceptance speech to the 1952 CIO convention, Reuther emphasised the need for unions to have a political dimension. However, his response to minority calls within the UAW for the creation of a third party was that, while the idea was laudable, Americans were not yet ready for it. His own socialist past was now never mentioned in UAW literature, and in the early 1950s he was careful to distance himself from his previous beliefs, telling the establishment figures of the Detroit Economic Club in 1953:

I felt in 1932 . . . that it [socialism] might be a better way to do things. I have long since stopped believing that Socialism is the answer . . . It's a fact that trade unions in general are showing resistance more than ever against moves towards Socialism . . . I believe in the free enterprise system as long as it demonstrates responsibility to the community. Government should only take on those projects that industry can't do and where it appears as a matter of necessity for government intervention.[21]

Yet at the same time he always recognised the value of radical political groupings able to feed fresh ideas into the labour movement. Organisations with socialist roots, such as the League for Industrial Democracy to which he had belonged as a student, and SANE, the anti-nuclear weapons campaigning organisation, were backed financially by the UAW and could usually expect Reuther's support. As Brendan Sexton, his friend and UAW colleague wrote, Reuther was different from the person that he had been in his twenties, but he was still in touch with his roots in the socialist movement and was anxious to appear morally acceptable to socialists around him, whom he counted upon to act as his 'conscience'.[22]

The optimistic assumptions of 1948 that the Democratic Party was capable of becoming the labour party of the US had suffered a reverse in congressional elections in 1950 when the UAW made a big effort to unseat Republican Senator Robert Taft in Ohio. Here the union was heavily rebuffed, provoking a further re-evaluation of its thinking. Once again the message seemed clear: that labour would have to settle for being just another minority group and would make progress only in conjunction with other minorities. During the 1950s Reuther's aim was to help realign the existing two main parties, working with the liberal wing of the Democratic Party with a view to radicalising policy, and hoping in the process to drive the conservative southern Democrats into their natural home among the Republicans. He was an enthusiastic supporter of Adlai Stevenson's presidential campaign in 1952 and, despite the latter's defeat, drew comfort from the fact that Democratic candidates did well in centres where the CIO was strong. Four years later, and against Meany's opposition, Reuther's intervention was important in winning AFL–CIO endorsement of Stevenson. By the late 1950s Reuther was beginning to feel that real progress towards a political realignment in the United States was being made. He told the British *Sunday Times* in June 1958 that the policies adopted by the Democratic Party at each convention were just as advanced as the British Labour Party's programme, and that American labour was just as radical as European labour. However, he was against the idea of the unions trying to capture the Democratic Party since to do so would be to destroy the broad base that was needed to make the party an effective instrument of policy.[23]

Reuther was now increasingly prominent in American politics and the right saw him as a dangerous threat to their interests. At the FBI, J. Edgar Hoover never wavered in his bizarre view that Reuther was a communist, despite the fact that in vetting him for membership of the Atomic Energy Commission in 1956, the FBI conducted 185 interviews with acquaintances, not one of whom could corroborate the allegations about Reuther's membership of the party. Between 1946 and 1953 the FBI file on Reuther swelled with 1,300 new references to him. In February of that year, even as he was proclaiming his willingness to work within the framework of free enterprise, Hoover intervened at the White House to ensure that Reuther was dropped from a list of names being considered for membership of the President's Committee on National Security. Three months later, Hoover lobbied to have him rejected for membership of the Marshall Plan agency's Public Advisory Board. And the following year an FBI officer was berated for briefing the White House on Reuther without disclosing all the details of his visit to the Soviet Union twenty years earlier.[24]

The FBI view jibed with that of the more virulent sections of the American right; both regarded Adlai Stevenson as a Reuther puppet. On the eve of the 1956 presidential election, an FBI *Digest of Communist Activities* observed: 'with Adlai Stevenson in the White House, the President of the United States would be under the dominant influence of Walter Reuther . . . With Reuther pulling the strings in Washington, the United States would take long strides towards a Fabian Socialist economy.'[25] During the same campaign the Committee of Constructive Conservatives issued a pamphlet written by Joseph P. Camp entitled *About the Man Who Will Win the 1956 Election*, which suggested that Reuther, rather than Stevenson, would be the winner in the event of a Democratic victory.

The anti-Reuther political campaign by business built up in 1957. The National Association of Manufacturers attacked him frequently, one issue of its journal in September 1957 containing three separate anti-Reuther pieces. Two months later the *Journal of Commerce* carried an editorial calling for the extension to the unions of anti-monopoly legislation for the purpose of 'stopping Reuther'. Before the 1958 congressional elections the Republicans constructed a 'fight the labour bosses' platform, with Reuther as target. The Committee for Constitutional Government was franking its mail with a stamp that said: 'Save the Republic and Stop Walter Reuther', and the Committee took a full page advertisement in the *Wall Street Journal* attacking the UAW leader.

The run-up to the 1958 election coincided with an intense Republican campaign to discredit organised labour through the hearings of the McClellan Senate Committee into union corruption. The activities of unions such as the Teamsters had provided the Republicans with their opportunity, but their hope was to extend the smear campaign to Reuther and the UAW. His main inquisitor on the committee was Republican Senator Barry Goldwater who told the Detroit Economic Club in January 1958: 'Walter Reuther and the UAW are a more dangerous menace than the sputniks or anything Russia might do.'[26] He had also been publicising a letter sent by Victor and Walter Reuther from Russia in 1934 which gave a glowing account of life in the USSR and allegedly concluded with the words, 'Carry on the fight for a Soviet America.' The letter had been written to Melvin Bishop whom Reuther later dismissed from his union post in 1947 and whom the Reuthers suspected of involvement in the attempted assassination of the UAW president in 1948. The letter had previously been published in at least six versions by groups seeking to discredit Reuther. His own position was that the offending words at the end of the letter were a forgery, and he insisted that the Senate Committee investigate the allegation. With the original document missing and Melvin Bishop proving to be an unsatisfactory witness, the Chairman, Senator McClellan, wrote to fellow Senator Hubert Humphrey: 'I think it is significant that, with the established unreliability of Mr Bishop and the fact that the existence and text of the letter were so questionable, no member of the committee saw fit to ask Mr Reuther any question about it.'[27]

Reuther himself gave evidence to the McClellan Committee for three days in March 1958. At the first session he opened with a lengthy statement berating the Republican members of the committee for their muckraking. The *Washington Post* reported: 'The red-haired labor leader held the Committee spellbound with a voluble 90-minute sermon on the obligations of Americans as citizens.' The report noted that as soon as he arrived, he promptly took charge of the senator's own hearing. The closing session ended with a shouting match between Reuther and Goldwater, the labour leader accusing the Republican and his associates of being in league to destroy him and the UAW. The focus of their concern, he said, was that as a union leader, he was too deeply involved in politics. He complained that for six months past, they had been engaged in a public campaign aimed at 'getting Reuther'.[28]

During the hearings, the Republicans had put the story about that Robert Kennedy, the committee's counsel, was afraid to investigate UAW finances for fear of upsetting the presidential aspirations of his brother, who was a member of the McClellan Committee. Reuther therefore insisted that his finances also be investigated, following which the committee's chief accountant reported on the union's frugal use of funds, the strict separation of personal from business items and the general scrupulousness of its accounting procedures. As the McClellan hearings finally closed in September 1959, Senator John Kennedy made a formal statement for the record:

> I think they [the hearings] have been a monumental misuse of time – for the members of the committee and for the persons directly involved . . . Apparently, none of the information was cross-checked or evaluated before it was broadcast from this committee . . . There has been nothing of consequence presented here that wasn't known more than a year and a half ago to this committee when the regular committee staff fully investigated these matters and recommended that the matter was not worthy of the committee's attention . . . I believe . . . it is a mistake for members of a Senate committee to use that committee to carry on political warfare against an organisation that they disapprove of.[29]

These hearings were the first close encounter between John Kennedy and Walter Reuther. Their relationship would be a significant element in American politics in the early 1960s.

Reuther's first major exposure to international trade union activities was through the Marshall Aid programme. From the outset, he had been a keen supporter of the Marshall Plan. Like many other trade unionists, he believed that it was capable of becoming a progressive programme, and in evidence to the Senate Foreign Relations Committee he called for labour to be granted a significant role in its administration. Yet when it became evident that the control of Marshall programmes was really in the hands of businessmen, CIO disillusionment grew, and by the early 1950s it was trying to develop its own approach to European reconstruction under which it would participate in aid programmes only if these dovetailed with its own trade union priorities. By 1951 the CIO had opened an office in Paris under the direction of Victor Reuther. The new CIO operation was conceived as a way of building the democratic trade union movement in Europe while avoiding the negative anti-communism of much of the AFL's activity. The AFL, through its Free Trade Union Committee directed by Jay Lovestone, believed in the need for a full-scale ideological war against communism – with a heavy emphasis on covert activities. In contrast, the CIO, especially under Reuther's leadership, stressed the importance of supporting democratic trade union organisation at the rank-and-file level and, by encouraging militant industrial activities, so helping the unions win majority support among workers.[30]

However, it was during this phase of the CIO's European operations that Reuther was drawn peripherally into the murky world of the Central Intelligence Agency when he received $50,000 from the Agency to finance union leadership training programmes being run by the International Confederation of Free Trade Unions (ICFTU) in France. The transaction was kept secret and came to light only fifteen years later in an exposé by a former CIA officer, Thomas Braden, who had passed him the money.[31] The disclosure was intended to embarrass Reuther at a time of intense UAW criticism of the AFL–CIO's links with the intelligence community; indeed, it did cause considerable disquiet among allies, who resented not just the fact that it had happened, but that it had been kept quiet for so long. The Reuther explanation is that the money was accepted in good faith with no awareness that it was from the CIA. That is quite possible: Victor Reuther had met Braden previously and had understood that he worked for the State Department or the Marshall Plan. Certainly the Reuther brothers were most careful in subsequent years to stay clear of CIA activities within the labour movement.[32]

On the other hand, Walter and Victor were undoubtedly prepared to accept American government and private foundation money for international trade union programmes, and this inevitably left them open to possible embarrassment. They were well aware of the danger. In 1948 Victor had suggested to Walter that the CIO seek such funding:

several top CIO people should meet with Truman and ask that federal funds . . . be made available to the CIO and AFL . . . I mean at least five million dollars . . . I cannot over-emphasize the importance [that] whatever funds are sent in the name of labor [are] channelled through trade union groups. Under no circumstances should there ever be any indication that funds other than trade union contributions are being sent to these trade union groups overseas.[33]

Although never crudely anti-communist in the way of the AFL, and while avoiding the entanglements with the CIA that were a central feature of AFL international work from the late 1940s, the CIO under Reuther was still strongly influenced by Cold War currents, and this was reflected in its willingness to take money from the US government for its international activities. In mitigation, one can point out that all major national trade union centres on both sides of the Iron Curtain had similar links.

Reuther became a member of the federal aid agency's Public Advisory Board in 1953, though the body was rarely convened, and labour movement disillusionment with the aid programme was now reaching a peak. This formative experience with the American aid programme in Europe greatly influenced his subsequent approach to international affairs. He was convinced of the need for liberal American trade unionists to be active overseas, presenting a positive, non-communist alternative vision to the negative Cold War postures adopted by the Eisenhower administration. However, he wanted this done in conjuction with the ICFTU, and in calling for the termination of separate CIO and AFL European activities, he was determined that American trade unions should follow an agreed policy within the framework of broad ICFTU programmes.

Relations between the AFL–CIO and the ICFTU became the principal focus of attention in the international field following the merger. At the founding conference of the ICFTU in London in 1950, Reuther had chaired the commission which drafted the organisation's Declaration of Principles – 'Bread, Peace and Freedom', and he was now keen that the ICFTU should pursue that statement vigorously. However, the business unionists of the old AFL were suspicious of the socialist-inclined Europeans who headed the ICFTU. George Meany, in particular, had a low opinion of the ICFTU's Dutch general secretary, J. H. Oldenbroek, whom he regarded as insufficiently anti-communist. From the early days of the ICFTU, the AFL had been an unenthusiastic affiliate, failing to pull its weight or to contribute its full financial share to ICFTU activities. Instead, it conducted its own independent international programme through Jay Lovestone's shadowy Free Trade Union Committee – what came to be known as 'Lovestoneism'. Despite commitments made during the merger negotiations to terminate this approach to international issues, the reunified AFL–CIO continued with its independent activities.

European trade union centres were resentful of AFL–CIO behaviour, and during the late 1950s there was much mutual suspicion and hostility between them and the Americans. Reuther was strongly opposed to Lovestoneism, and during these years he spent much time and energy trying to secure AFL–CIO compliance with its own official policy of working through the ICFTU, while at the same time he attempted to mediate between the AFL–CIO and its European critics. The major substantive disagreement between the AFL–CIO and the ICFTU was over the question of how best to approach the development of the trade union movement in Africa. On this issue, conflicting views about the dangers of communism, colonialism and Pan Africanism came together. The AFL–CIO wanted a more vigorous anti-communist programme than the ICFTU seemed set to deliver, but they were also much more determined opponents of colonialism than were their European counterparts, and therefore willing to support Pan Africanism. In turn, these disagreements over policy in Africa spilled over into a debate about the adequacy of Oldenbroek's leadership of the ICFTU.

Reuther worked both sides of the fence in this debate, opposing the AFL–CIO's free-wheeling interventionism in Africa, but also showing his concern that the ICFTU was bureaucratic and too slow-moving. In trying to galvanise the Confederation into more dynamic action, he supported the election of Swedish metalworkers' union leader, Arne Geijer, to the presidency of the ICFTU. The two men had similar views on politics and trade unionism and were to develop a close personal relationship. Meanwhile, in discussions with Kenyan labour leader, Tom Mboya, in the spring of 1959 Reuther was persuaded that the ICFTU strategy in Africa risked failure. Subsequently, at a meeting between Reuther and Geijer in Sweden in May 1959, the two hatched a plan to remove Oldenbroek from his post as general secretary. It was a ruthless power play, as he himself recognised, but he justified it on the grounds that it was not an attempt to capture control of the Confederation but rather to free it from the domination of the general secretary.[34] As long as Oldenbroek remained in office, Meany had an excuse for continuing the AFL–CIO's separate and divisive international activities. In these circumstances, Reuther's opposition to Oldenbroek was calculated to save the ICFTU from the damage that further autonomous AFL–CIO activities might cause.

> Following their Swedish meeting, Reuther wrote to Geijer:
> I feel very strongly about this matter, for in the absence of the ICFTU becoming an adequate, dynamic force there is no possible other force that can counteract the forces of Communism . . . we cannot continue to permit the domination of the ICFTU by the inflexible personality of Oldenbroek . . . The hour is much later than we realize, and I share the belief that the people of Asia, Africa and Latin America who are on the march will not wait nor adjust their time schedule to accommodate Mr Oldenbroek's inflexible attitude. The direction that these hundreds of millions of people in these three critical areas will take will in large measure depend on the kind of practical aid we can give them in building effective, democratic trade union forces . . . If we do not act at the December Congress, then we might forfeit our opportunity. History will not wait.[35]

Eventually Oldenbroek was eased out of his position in 1960, but the ICFTU was bloodied as a result of the internal struggle, the AFL–CIO leadership appeared no more ready to work within the ICFTU, and for Reuther the task remained of persuading his American colleagues that a new team of officers in the ICFTU would make the organisation worthy of support.

The second string to Reuther's international bow, and ultimately a more productive field of operations than the ICFTU, was his work within the International Metalworkers' Federation (IMF). He first made contact with the IMF soon after being elected UAW president in 1946 when its Swiss general secretary, Konrad Ilg, sought him out as a likely ally against communism. Ilg explained that the Federation was distinct from the communist-influenced World Federation of Trade Unions in its strategy, being more concerned with basic trade union issues.[36] Along with a number of other American unions, the UAW affiliated to the IMF in 1949, the Americans by then comprising almost half the total membership. Reuther secured a seat on the executive board and was elected president of the IMF's newly-formed automotive committee in 1950.

With a strong American presence in the IMF, there was a change of emphasis in strategy towards a more pragmatic pursuit of improvements through collective bargaining and away from the continental union predilection for staking out theoretical positions in the class war and then relying on lobbying government over legislative reform of working conditions. The American Fordist influence was also reflected in a new trade union concern for increasing production and buying power. Reuther was an enthusiast for this change: 'For the first time we have a genuine attempt to develop a practical collective bargaining program, and to get away from the abstract, theoretical approach heretofore characterizing most international trade union conferences.'[37]

UAW influence within the IMF extended beyond the fact of Reuther's membership of the executive board. Their considerable financial input and the close interest that Walter took in the Federation's affairs through his brother Victor, the head of the UAW's international programme, meant that in practice the general secretary, Adolph Graedel, took few important decisions without first obtaining UAW approval. The Reuthers were free with their advice to him, and it was often difficult to distinguish between advice and instructions. Reuther worked hard to ensure that trusted people were in the top jobs. He lobbied enthusiastically on behalf of German metalworkers' union leader, Otto Brenner, for the vacant presidency of the IMF in 1960, happier to work with him than his conservative British rival for the post, AEU president William Carron. And when IMF assistant general secretary Charles Levinson, whose salary was supplemented by the UAW, began to steer a course independent of UAW interests, Reuther brought pressure to have him removed from his post.

Three areas of IMF policy were of particular interest to Reuther in the 1950s – France/Italy, Japan and Mexico. In each case the IMF project was to help build non-communist trade unionism at the grass roots or to try to concert the activities of separate metalworker unions by bringing them into the IMF fold. In these geographical areas, the UAW undertook to make a special financial contribution or supplied key personnel to administer the programme. IMF activity in France and Italy was an outgrowth of Marshall Plan labour programmes. Reuther was the chief instigator of a secret fund subscribed to by some of the larger IMF affiliates, from which subventions were made to the non-communist metalworking unions in those two countries. The UAW provided about a fifth of the total funding, and the long-term outcome was to help create a radical and democratic alternative to the French communists in the form of the CFTC/CFDT in the 1960s, and more significantly to contribute to the 'turn to the left' in 1960s Italian politics.[38] In Mexico and Japan, where cheap labour was beginning to threaten autoworkers' jobs in the USA, the IMF aim was to try to overcome divisions among metalworking unions and thereby render them more effective forces for collective bargaining. In Japan, Reuther was anxious to resist what he called the 'traditional and illogical high tariff approach to the problem'. And he provided a $10,000 grant to enable the IMF to send a representative to the country in 1956 on a six-month exploratory mission to assess the scope for IMF organising. When IMF activities began in Mexico the following year, a Reuther supporter, Dan Benedict, was put in charge of a $20,000 assistance programme to develop union organisation and leadership.

Though Reuther never sought to develop an international programme independent of the ICFTU and IMF, the UAW did conduct extensive activities abroad, directed by Victor Reuther, which aimed to complement the work of the two international bodies to which they were affiliated. At one level the range of Reuther's interests reflected his awareness of the need to counter, wherever possible, the influence of Lovestoneism backed by CIA funds. Jay Lovestone was waging a global ideological war against communism. To Reuther, with his primary concern to improve living conditions and self-organisation at the grass roots, this focus was ill-conceived and wasteful. It was from this perspective that he intervened personally or deployed the resources of the UAW to influence labour movement politics in countries as different as Ghana, Finland, Cuba and Tunisia at various times in the late 1950s.

Reuther was always conscious of the need to present a democratic alternative to communism yet, under Eisenhower's foreign policy, the non-communist left everywhere was being ignored by the USA. In 1956–7 he engaged Adolph Sturmthal, the veteran secretary of the pre-war Socialist International, and currently the holder of a UAW-endowed chair at Roosevelt University, Chicago to make an extensive tour of Western Europe and to report on political developments. In particular Reuther wanted him to assess what activities the UAW and like-minded sections of American labour might undertake in order to influence European politics in a progressive direction. Reuther was especially concerned to discover the significance of the pressures for change that were building up in German Social Democracy, and he was interested in exploring the possibilities of helping to advance the much-discussed 'opening to the left' in Italian politics. [39] His overseas interests were the clearest indication of his belief that freedom and democracy were indivisible and that autoworkers in Detroit would benefit in the long run from improvements in economic and social conditions of workers in other countries. His international idealism was genuine, and though pressure of commitments at home sometimes constrained his work in this field, the truth was that he was a 'doer' where other union leaders were content to pass resolutions.

His own most ambitious foreign excursion was to India in 1956 where he had been invited by the national trade union centre, INTUC. He visited the country against the background of deteriorating US–Indian relations and recent allegations by George Meany that India's foreign policy was aiding the USSR and China. Following the Geneva Conference, the USSR had just embarked on an aid programme to developing countries, and American hostility was now visited upon the recipients. As well as countering the hostility that had recently been directed at India in the USA, Reuther's hope was to build links with the Indian labour movement, ease INTUC fears that ICFTU activities in India were being pursued in the interests of US foreign policy, urge greater unity among the divided Indian unions, staunch communist attempts to promote an 'independent' federation of Asian unions, and give support to a form of trade unionism that relied more on industrial activities and collective bargaining and less on political patronage.

While in the subcontinent, he announced his opposition to the current military emphasis of US foreign aid in Asia, 85 per cent of which was for arms procurement. He observed at a meeting of MPs in the Indian Parliament that much of the country's budget was going on guns because of their fear of Pakistan, which was in turn being armed by the United States. Indian people did not want American guns to *defend* their condition, he argued, rather they wanted to *change* it. These anti-militarist, anti-colonial sentiments were very different from the crude anti-communism that Indians had been used to hearing from the USA. Reuther was received as an international statesman and had discussions with leading political figures. In meetings with Prime Minister Pandit Nehru, he was told that the US had refused aid to India's developing metal industries and that the USSR had now stepped in with assistance. Reuther was anxious to see the US enter that field also. Indian steel industry technicians, he believed, should be trained in the United States, and as a direct result of his pressure the Ford Foundation later financed a programme under which over 200 Indian technicians were brought to the USA for training.⁴⁰ On his return to the United States, he briefed Secretary of State John Foster Dulles and reported on his visit to the Senate Foreign Relations Committee, arguing the case for $1bn. in aid for the country over the course of her second five-year plan. More generally, he proposed that American aid be given to all free Third World countries, not just those that were aligned to the USA.

Reuther was greatly excited by his Indian visit and the possibilities that he saw for various forms of inter-governmental and trade union co-operation. It had been his intention to return to the country in 1957 or 1958 but, over-committed as ever, he was unable to do so and the promise of some of the initiatives that his trip prompted, such as the movement to rationalise the Indian trade union structure and the hopes for a major trade union exchange programme with the Americans was not sustained. His own enthusiasm could not compensate for the negative attitude of the Eisenhower administration to India, and the weaknesses of the Indian trade union movement were of a magnitude that the ICFTU could not overcome.

In the year following his trip to India, he was the AFL–CIO fraternal delegate to the annual conference of the British Trades Union Congress at Blackpool and made an extraordinary impact with a typical speech in which he urged the deployment of technology to benefit people, putting peace first, and going beyond negative anti-communism. 'Too often,' he said, 'the policies of the free world are shaped in the image of our fears and our hatreds. I believe it is time that the free world begin to shape its policies in the images of its hopes and its aspirations and its common faith. It is time to begin to fight as hard for the things we believe in, as we fight in opposition to the things to which we are opposed.' The British press gave him a rapturous reception. The *Sunday Times* reported: 'Throughout the Congress . . . one man spoke like a . . . prophet – and his was the Voice of America.' The *Daily Herald* enthused:

> The spellbinder from Detroit, the Pied Piper of Hope, excited this conference today with an explosion of vitality as American as a skyscraper and as adventurous as a covered wagon . . . He gave us the American dream, the

dawn of the era when we have the tools of unprecedented abundance, when social justice and peace and plenty are inseparable and are there for the taking . . . Reuther is a 20th century pedlar who backs his dreams with the reality of Detroit and Pittsburgh, atomic power and automation.

'Reuther's Day' was how the *Daily Express* reporter described it. 'No overseas visitor in living memory has made such an immense impact by his personality and his tempestuous oratory.' The *News Chronicle* correspondent reported that it was 'one of the most dazzling pieces of oratory I have ever heard . . . In future years TUC veterans will say to each other: "Do you remember the 1957 congress . . . the day that Walter Reuther made that speech?" ' And the *Socialist Digest* noted that if you were looking for a way of describing the congress, there was no better way than to say it was 'the Walter Reuther Congress'. 'No fraternal delegate has ever made such an impact on a TUC. And few men, even in our own Labour Movement, can have succeeded so well in capturing the imagination of the Congress within the limits of a 35 minute speech . . . But Walter Reuther is a remarkable man.'[41]

Reuther really came of age as an international figure in 1959, the year in which he had talks with Soviet leaders, Deputy Prime Minister Anastas Mikoyan and Party Secretary Nikita Khrushchev and was invited by Willy Brandt to address a May Day rally of German workers in Berlin. He met Mikoyan over lunch in Washington in January 1959 along with four other union leaders. Reuther dominated the proceedings which developed into a vigorous exchange between himself and the Soviet leader. He questioned Mikoyan sharply about Soviet international policies. In particular, he asked why Germany could not be reunited with free elections. As they debated the meaning of democracy, Mikoyan remarked that there was no difference between the Democratic and Republican parties in the USA, but Reuther stopped him short with the observation that there were more programmatic differences between the two American parties than there had been between the Bolsheviks and Mensheviks at the time of their split.[42]

Back in Moscow, Mikoyan reported that his rudest reception in the USA had been at the hands of Reuther.[43] However, the well-publicised exchange made him a hero in other parts, and German workers in particular flocked to hear him when three months later in Berlin he was a speaker at the Berlin May Day Rally alongside Mayor

Willy Brandt. Over half a million Berliners turned out to hear them, the biggest post-war rally in the city. The son of German immigrants, Reuther reminded them that he had been in Berlin in 1933 when Hitler came to power and had been active in Berlin affairs again in the 1940s, speaking out on behalf of German reconstruction and supporting the airlift. There could be no peace in Germany without reunification and he called on Berliners to stand fast for they did not stand alone. His message was directed as much at those in East Germany, and he pointed out that while Soviet workers had made great progress and had won more bread, they still lacked freedom. Yet workers everywhere wanted both bread and freedom. East Berliners were not allowed to attend the rally, but in the afternoon the border guards relaxed controls and Reuther and Brandt jointly addressed over 20,000 East Berliners in an amphitheatre on the outskirts of the city.

Reuther's encounter with Mikoyan was only a trial run for a more celebrated meeting with Khrushchev in San Francisco in September 1959. The Soviet leader had hoped for a chance to address the AFL–CIO convention then in session in the city, but Meany refused to appear in the same room as him. Reuther, however, believed that it was always worth speaking with opponents, and certainly the propaganda opportunity should not be squandered. So he made private arrangements for the meeting with Khrushchev, Andrei Gromyko and the novelist Mikhail Sholokhov at the Mark Hopkins Hotel and was accompanied by only a handful of fellow union leaders. In fact, the event was carefully arranged, Reuther had been well briefed by organisations such as the American Jewish Committee on questions that he might ask and answers that might be given, and a press conference for 300 newspaper reporters was scheduled afterwards.

With Reuther again acting as spokesman for the American group, the meeting was rather more bad-tempered than the one with Mikoyan. Over more than three hours, the two sides sparred and at times traded insults on matters of international politics and ideology. Khrushchev refused to discuss self-determination for the people of Eastern Europe. He became belligerent and banged the table when asked about the Hungarian uprising and spoke of it as the work of hooligans and saboteurs, saying that Imry Nagy was a fascist. When Reuther suggested that trade unions in the USSR were under management control, Khrushchev countered that the American organisations were 'capitalist lackeys'. Reuther asked him about Soviet censorship, at which Khrushchev stood up, gave a hilarious impersonation of a can-can dancer that he had seen on a Hollywood set some days before and suggested that such immoral displays should be censored. When asked by Reuther if the Soviet press would publish a speech of his, Khrushchev said yes, if it was constructive – whereupon the labour leader quickly handed him the text of his May Day speech in Berlin.

Reuther was keen to milk the episode for its propaganda value and an English- and Russian-language transcript of the meeting was subsequently published by the Freedom Fund entitled 'Khrushchev and the American Unions'.[44] Reuther gave interviews to *émigré* journalists whose reports circulated in the Soviet bloc, creating a big impression in East Germany and Berlin. Meanwhile the Soviet authorities were keen to discredit him, the trade union newspaper *Trud* attacking him and reporting the existence of his abandoned Russian 'wife'.[45] Khrushchev's own feelings about Reuther were not in doubt. At a meeting with President Kennedy in 1961, he spoke of America being controlled by monopolists, at which point Kennedy reminded him that he had met Reuther. 'Yes,' replied Khrushchev, 'I met him. We hung the likes of Reuther in Russia in 1917.'[46] It was perhaps an interesting comment on Reuther that a contemporary cartoon showed Khrushchev and Goldwater with arms linked saying, 'I hate Walter Reuther.'

The 1950s saw Reuther in his prime. He had established undisputed control of the UAW and made it the most influential of unions, untainted by the corruption that affected a number of other labour organisations. As CIO president he had helped reunite the labour movement in the hope that it would play a more significant role in American society. Within the AFL–CIO he had established himself as the acknowledged leader of the liberal wing and was busy promoting his progressive views within the wider movement. As a negotiator, he had been responsible for a sequence of path-breaking agreements in the first half of the decade. His approach to collective negotiations was eversensitive to the interplay between national economic management and the agenda of the bargaining table, and in this field he regularly established the yardsticks by which other trade unions would measure their achievements. Yet as the decade progressed and it became harder to emulate the bargaining achievements of the early 1950s, Reuther also came up against the issue of recurrent rank and file disquiet over the nature and pace of change at work and the intractable problem of how to protect workers in this situation while maintaining organisational discipline. Politically he had hitched his wagon to the Democratic Party while hoping for a realignment of the two main parties. His political interests gave him the appearance of being among the most powerful figures in the United States, and as such he became a prime target for the far right. More than any other labour leader, he was increasingly active in international affairs – in an ill-starred attempt to establish the ICFTU as a powerful force, with more success helping to build a solid international organisation of metalworking unions, and with boundless energy taking his own distinct trade union message to countries as far apart as Mexico and India. Though an international statesman of stature, he felt increasingly blocked at home in the years of drift under Eisenhower. A political change was needed to break the logjam, and by 1960 Reuther's hopes were firmly pinned on the promise of John F. Kennedy.

6 Reuther and the New Frontier

John F. Kennedy had no more committed supporter than Walter Reuther. In the mid–1950s the UAW president had been less than impressed with Kennedy's record on civil rights and had lectured him: 'Young man, when you change your voting record, then I'll support you.' However, his respect for the Massachussetts Senator had grown during the McClellan hearings, and at the 1960 Democratic Convention Reuther backed his candidacy for President, preferring him over long-time political allies Hubert Humphrey and Adlai Stevenson. After the convention, Reuther returned with Kennedy to Hyannisport at the beginning of August 1960 and spent some days there discussing policy and staffing of a future administration. It was there, for example, that Reuther sold Kennedy on the idea of the Peace Corps. The UAW subsequently threw all its effort into the Democratic Party campaign: Reuther travelled with the Senator on a number of occasions and shared platforms with him. Walter's brother, Roy, also took leave of absence from his UAW post to become a co-director of the Democrats' 1960 voter registration drive. A year into his presidency, Kennedy received a rousing welcome at the 1962 UAW convention. He told the assembled autoworkers: 'Last week, after speaking to the Chambers of Commerce and the Presidents of the American Medical Association, I began to wonder how I got elected. And now I remember.'[1]

Hopes were high for the reforming policies of the new administration in domestic and international fields. The arrival of the new President unleashed a mass of creative energy in Reuther. The New Frontier, Alliance for Progress, trade liberalisation and talk of a Decade of Development were ideas that chimed with his own interests, and in the coming years he was appointed to a number of government policy advisory bodies such as the Presidential Advisory Committee on Labor–Management Policy; the President's Committee on Equal Employment Opportunity; the Labor Advisory Committee to the Alliance for Progress; the Public Advisory Committee for Trade Negotiations, and the National Commission on Technology, Automation and Economic Progress. The anti-poverty and civil rights programmes seemed to map a way forward from the social neglect of the Eisenhower years, and Reuther would be an enthusiastic supporter of both. More generally, his hope was that the change of administration would improve the economic climate for labour, since the election had been largely fought around rival claims about real and potential rates of economic growth.

Reuther tried hard to influence the new administration's economic policy, but there were important differences between what the UAW expected of Kennedy and the influential views being pushed by another member of the Kennedy circle, J. K. Galbraith. Galbraith's 'affluent society' thesis boiled down to a series of policy propositions: that the US had an excessive preoccupation with the production of private goods which squeezed out necessary production for public use; and that a sufficient level of private production could be maintained with a lower level of employment, which in turn would reduce inflationary pressures. Reuther rejected the Galbraith line and argued for a much greater commitment to economic growth. He maintained that there were still many unmet needs, both private and public, and that the country had the capacity to provide for both so long as policies of growth were pursued. At the heart of his philosophy was the notion that higher wages were necessary to overcome poverty and furnish the consumer spending that would drive the economy to higher levels of economic growth. Inflation, Reuther maintained, was basically a product of administered pricing.[2]

In economic policy, the Kennedy administration never quite lived up to the hopes that labour had for it. By 1962 UAW members were becoming disillusioned, and Reuther warned that the President risked defeat if unemployment were not reduced.[3] He opposed Kennedy's call for wage restraint, and complained over the failure of the federal government to develop tripartite machinery that would facilitate a rational debate about economic priorities. Deeply influenced by the practice of European social democracy, Reuther was a persistent advocate of democratic economic planning through which private economic decisions could be harmonised with public policy. In defence policy, too, he was disappointed and as a supporter of disarmament was forced to swallow the President's resumption of nuclear testing in

1962. Yet there was little he could do to change this, given his strategy of cultivating the Democratic establishment.

Reuther was conscious of the tightrope he had to walk in dealing with the administration. 'What the labor movement has got to do,' he argued, 'is try to find a way to . . . have a working relationship with the Establishment – because it bargains with the Establishment . . . It can't pretend the Establishment doesn't exist and it can't act as though it has no contact with it . . . But the labor movement ought not to become absorbed in the Establishment.'⁴ Ready access to the White House could be a great advantage, but it is not at all clear whether it was a case of Reuther exercising influence on the administration or vice versa. As the columnist Murray Kempton observed: 'it is the posture of the American labor movement to disagree with a decision of President Kennedy's only up to the point that it is made.' Reuther had nowhere else to go, and in the process was drawn from the left to the centre of the Democratic Party, his ambition of a political realignment in America reduced to a programme of political adjustment.⁵

Another matter where Kennedy failed to move quickly enough for Reuther was in the field of civil rights. Reuther began to focus on the issue in spring 1963 when he led 125,000 people on a Freedom Walk down Woodward Avenue in Detroit – the largest civil rights march to date – and then addressed the rally at Cobo Hall with Martin Luther King. That same spring the UAW donated $160,000 to help bail out NAACP civil rights marchers gaoled in Birmingham, Alabama. He committed himself fully to the civil rights cause in the tense summer of 1963, writing to Attorney General Robert Kennedy that it would be the priority item in the period ahead. He was instrumental in building a broad-based coalition of church and labour leaders aimed at publicising the cause,⁶ and in the famous March on Washington on 28 August he was the leading non-black speaker.

The event, to commemorate the Proclamation of Emancipation in 1863, was meant to be a march for jobs, focusing on the economic side of civil rights to which neither King nor his colleagues gave high priority. Reuther was the obvious labour leader to speak on this theme. He told the huge crowd that the Kennedy civil rights legislation was a modest first step which needed strengthening, especially in the area of fair employment provisions: 'The job question is crucial because we will not solve the problems of education or housing, or public accommodations as long as millions of American Negroes are treated as second class economic citizens . . . And so our slogan has got to be "fair employment" but fair employment within the framework of full employment so that every American can have a job.' Civil rights, he said, was a moral question which transcended party politics, and the march was the first step in a total effort to mobilise the moral conscience of America.[7] He had failed to secure AFL–CIO support for the march: indeed, Meany had tried to block labour participation. However, Reuther was determined to demonstrate his own liberal credentials, and was saddened that the entire American labour movement had not participated. After the march, blacks and liberal whites worked together better than ever. At the 1964 UAW convention Reuther announced the creation of the Citizen's Crusade Against Poverty with a budget of $1 million, out of which would come the 1966 Poor People's Convention, focusing on the problems of the working poor. He also assigned 100 members to work with Martin Luther King on a voter registration drive in Chicago.

Reuther had been much enamoured of his special relationship with Kennedy, and after the President was assassinated was determined to retain access to the Johnson White House, despite the fact that Johnson, as Senate majority leader, had sustained the southern filibuster of progressive legislation. In 1960 Reuther had opposed the choice of the Texas Senator as Kennedy's running mate, but before Kennedy's funeral Johnson phoned and told him: 'My friend, I need your friendship and support now more than ever before.'[8] Reuther subsequently developed a particularly close rapport with Johnson and became a frequent visitor to the White House, so much so that right-wing commentators were disturbed at his ease of access. Ironically, in this apparently privileged position, he was still under investigation by the FBI for his sponsorship of the NAACP and SANE.

Access to Johnson carried a price, and Reuther was forced to sacrifice some of his standing in the field of civil rights to maintain his position as an insider. The occasion was the 1964 Democratic Party convention and the dispute over the attempt to seat the integrated delegates of the Mississippi Freedom Democratic Party (supported by the Student Nonviolent Co-ordinating Committee (SNCC)) in place of the all-white official delegation from Mississippi. It was an episode that demonstrated how little room for manoeuvre Reuther had while allied to the Democratic establishment. Before the convention, SNCC had approached Reuther to support their tactic, but he declined, sensing that this might lead to a confrontation with Lyndon Johnson. For a time, though, he did allow UAW legal counsel Joe Rauh to work for the SNCC cause.

President Johnson's approach was to ask black groups for a moratorium on aggressive civil rights tactics in the build-up to the presidential election. King, A. Philip Randolph and other leaders agreed, but not the SNCC, and Reuther now pressed Rauh to withdraw from the campaign. At the convention Johnson essayed a compromise under which two token MFDP delegates would be seated, with a promise that no non-integrated delegations would be admitted in future. Hubert Humphrey, a vice-presidential hopeful, was given the task of selling the deal, and in this he enlisted the support of Reuther, who left off contract negotiations to assist. Rauh, who referred to this as 'Reuther's dirty job', generously conceded that the UAW president was motivated by a determination to remain on good terms with the President for the positive benefits that it might bring his members and the less well-off.[9] In this case, part of the prize was to clinch the vice-presidential nomination for the pro-labour Hubert Humphrey. However, Johnson's compromise was not accepted by the SNCC, the gap between the more militant black activists and white liberals now widened, and Reuther's opponents viewed the episode as clear evidence of the fact that he would barter principles for political expediency. Critics claimed that his brand of practical liberalism stirred few hearts among the civil rights activists of the 1960s. They regarded him only as a distant sympathiser,[10] though in truth he was still the outstanding liberal voice of his generation among American trade unionists.

In the American automobile industry, production was again booming by 1963. Yet unemployment persisted, and Reuther focused on measures of job creation for the 1964 round of collective bargaining, fearing that the growing right-wing forces of Senator Barry Goldwater might capitalise on the disaffection of a permanent economic underclass. Profit-sharing again featured prominently in his thinking, not so much with a view to putting cash in members' pockets, but as a device for accumulating the necessary funds to finance shorter hours, early retirement and the various social benefits on the union's agenda. Although the corporations fiercely resisted this proposal, economic benefits were readily affordable and conceded by the employers at the bargaining table, including measures that would create more jobs. 'Technological Progress Without Fear' was how the union trumpeted the gains, among them the principle of early retirement at sixty and additional vacation entitlement. Innovative benefits provided for firms to pay tuition costs for workers undertaking a personal study programme related to their employment. Reuther's social idealism was also reflected in a clause under which workers could volunteer for service in the Peace Corps without loss of seniority and with full re-employment rights on completing their two years of service.

However, the real battle in 1964 was over the move to humanise the workplace and curb speed-up. Complaints about increasingly heavy workloads were once again a prominent issue, with the return to high levels of production. Symptomatic of this was the fact that in 1963 over one-third of officers in UAW production locals had been defeated in bids for re-election, largely because of their failure to protect members adequately in this regard. Reuther began to talk about the industry's 'gold-plated sweatshops',[11] and the UAW was determined to oppose management practices that affronted human dignity, such as closed-circuit television surveillance and monitoring of workers by machine recording devices. It took local strike action by over 350,000 workers at 130 GM locations in September–October 1964 and costing the union over $40 million in strike pay to secure some qualitative improvements in the prison-like atmosphere which continued to pervade many of the company's plants. Both sides represented the outcome as a victory. Reuther claimed that 'no strike in the history of our union . . . has yielded the kind of meaningful results . . . as this strike.' But GM's president insisted: 'We haven't agreed to anything that is going to impair our responsibility to our shareholders to run an efficient business . . . and that's what this strike has been about.'[12] The quality of working life was now on the agenda, but it was still not the case that Reuther's approach to bargaining allowed sufficient workers' control at the point of production.

Reuther met President Johnson soon after his landslide election victory in 1964, to urge a bold approach to the concept of the 'Great Society'. The policies of the early 1960s had been an advance on those of Eisenhower, but had only produced a small reduction in the intolerably high level of unemployment. The single most important need was a significant increase in federal spending. The 'Great Society' could not be built on market forces and the administration should begin to influence private sector decisions by publishing its own projections for economic growth.[13] Valued as they were, the anti-poverty and integrationist policies of the Great Society only scratched the surface of the problem, in Reuther's view.

As inflation increased in the mid–1960s, fuelled by the economic strains imposed by the Vietnam War, Reuther found himself increasingly at odds with Johnson's policies for wage restraint. Guideposts for wage increases were being applied mechanistically, without regard to increasing productivity. However, unlike Meany, whose opposition to the government guideposts simply reflected the business unionist's resistance to all interference with free collective bargaining, Reuther was concerned with the inequity of the measures and the fact that they did not go far enough. In 1966 he told fellow members of the President's Labor Management Advisory Committee that labour could not take seriously the anti-inflationary policy when it was directed only at wages and not at prices and profits. It was also his view that anti-inflationary policies must not override basic commitments to full employment, especially when the rate of joblessness in the United States was double the average for Europe. What he called for was a fully-fledged prices and incomes policy to cover all forms of income, such as appeared to be the objective of European social democrats, most recently the British Labour Party. Yet what seemed possible in Europe was beyond the limits of practical politics in the USA. And despite his efforts to expunge from the vocabulary of professional economists the notion of a 'wage–price spiral' (he talked of the 'profit–price–wage spiral'), he was fighting a losing battle.[14]

Whatever hope Reuther may have nursed that relations within the AFL–CIO would gradually improve was dispelled in the early 1960s. The optimistic view had been that problems arose because of the way things were done, rather than as a result of insurmountable differences in policy. The AFL–CIO, sympathetic observers said, had simply inherited the craft wing's deep-seated tradition of centralised leadership, which tended to exclude local leaders and members from democratic decision-making. However, the problem went deeper, and major policy differences in domestic and international affairs contributed to the growing tension between Meany and Reuther in the early 1960s. Reuther was angered over Meany's lack of support for the organising drive among migrant farm labourers in California, and in foreign affairs at the continued evidence that Lovestone was determining aspects of international policy 'on the hoof'. Disconsolate at the deteriorating relations between the craft and industrial wings of the AFL–CIO in spring 1961, he told a senior ICFTU staff member that, despite the merger, 'we have been united in name only'.[15] Was the apparent price of unity – a conservative, bureaucratic labour movement – too high to pay?

In practice the AFL–CIO continued to wage war on the ICFTU, even after, with Meany's support, Oldenbroek was replaced in 1960 as general secretary by the Belgian, Omer Becu. The revitalisation of the Confederation depended very much on adequate funding in the years ahead, and especially on financial contributions from the Americans, the largest and best-endowed affiliate. Yet Meany soon parted company with Becu when efforts to place Lovestone's close colleague, Irving Brown, in the post of assistant general secretary were rejected. Denouncing the ICFTU as a 'cesspool', and expressing a personal preference for withdrawal, Meany at first refused to pay over outstanding dues, and then ensured that American contributions in the next few years were so limited as to face the ICFTU with a perpetual funding crisis.[16] International organising efforts by the Confederation were crippled, while the much-resented independent activities by the AFL–CIO in Africa and Latin America continued. Reuther wrote to Meany that he was 'particularly saddened by the depth of your personal bitterness towards the ICFTU and its leadership . . . it is as unthinkable that the AFL–CIO should withdraw from the ICFTU, as for the US to withdraw from the UN.'[17]

The outstanding instance of the AFL–CIO ploughing its own furrow in international affairs was in Latin America through the American Institute for Free Labor Development (AIFLD), a creation of the Federation through which government and industry helped finance trade union developmental policy under the Alliance for Progress. AIFLD was created in 1961 to provide training in the United States for Latin American union leaders and to develop social programmes for workers' housing, co-operatives and credit unions there. With an annual budget of over $1 million, rising by the mid–1960s to $5 million, the Institute's main financial backer was the US government through the Agency for International Development (AID). From the very beginning, the presence of businessmen on the AIFLD board suggested that a basic objective of the programme in Latin America was to secure the development of a pro-management trade union movement.

Reuther was invited to join the AIFLD board in late 1961 when the form and thrust of the Institute had already been decided. IMF affiliates in Latin America believed it unwise of him to be identified with a body that included among its directors Peter Grace of W. R. Grace & Company, a corporation with extensive Latin American interests and a reputation for anti-unionism and support for military dictatorships in the southern hemisphere. Victor Reuther cautioned him to be wary and urged him to challenge Meany on the role of AIFLD and the composition of its board. In fact, Reuther played no direct role in the affairs of AIFLD but, in the interests of AFL–CIO harmony, fought shy of a direct confrontation with Meany. Yet as Victor pointed out, it was a fragile merger indeed if it could not withstand a clear choice between serving the interests of workers and being used as a company union tool for major corporations in their effort to secure pliable trade unions.[18]

By 1964 it was evident that AIFLD was playing an increasingly prominent part in the domestic politics of Latin America. AIFLD-trained trade unionists had been prominent in the CIA-financed general strike that toppled the Jagan government in British Guiana and had been involved in the military coup that brought down the Goulart regime in Brazil. The communist movement was beginning to make capital out of this embarrassing association of the American labour movement with what, in effect, was developing into an extended arm of CIA intelligence gathering. '[Y]ou will understand why, as a trade unionist, I feel a sense of revulsion,' Victor wrote to his brother,[19] while continuing to urge steps to end the association with the Institute.

Eventually, in 1965 Reuther took a stand over the unsavoury business connection with AIFLD when he learned that a Grace plant in Towanda, New York had issued anti-union leaflets to defeat a UAW organising campaign, one of them carrying the message: 'In Grace plants no-one needs a union partner in his pay envelope.' He resigned from AIFLD on the instructions of the UAW executive board in September 1965, though it seems that the decision was taken after much deliberation and with some misgiving that it would further damage relations within the AFL–CIO.

As relations between Reuther and Meany deteriorated in the early 1960s on a range of issues big and small, the latter increasingly sought to marginalise the autoworkers' leader within the AFL–CIO and frustrate his efforts to wield influence further afield. Meany refused to accept a

Reuther-supported nominee for a vacant seat on the IUD, Reuther's own bailiwick. He blocked Reuther's attempt to have his former trusted assistant, Jack Conway, appointed to the vacant post of Under Secretary of Labour. He vetoed a proposal from Adlai Stevenson that Kennedy appoint Reuther to succeed him as a member of the United States delegation to the United Nations, an honour much coveted by Reuther. He disputed Reuther's right to speak to Kennedy on behalf of the AFL–CIO on an urgent matter of economic policy, despite his being the chairman of the Federation's Economic Policy Committee. Meany chose not to submit the UAW president's name among a list of people to serve on the Federal Labor Department's International Affairs Committee, despite his being the most active person in the field. He opposed important aspects of Reuther's international work. In petty fashion, he even snubbed the UAW president by keeping him off the escort party for Kennedy when the President attended the 1961 AFL–CIO convention, and refused to allow Reuther to accept an invitation to appear with him on a television programme to mark the fiftieth anniversary of the Labor Department.

There was a clear struggle between the two men for the ear of the President. Kennedy certainly had a rapport with Reuther and likened his personal difficulties with Meany to those that he himself had in dealings with de Gaulle. However, the most important consideration for the President was that he had been elected with a tiny majority, could not afford to alienate the AFL–CIO, and therefore let it be known that Meany was to be recognised as labour's sole authorised ambassador to the US government.

For all the promise of the Kennedy age, Reuther's domestic standing had fallen in the early 1960s. Hopes of revitalising the labour movement at home were turning sour, and while Reuther was highly critical of the conservative leadership of Meany – he was a man who boasted that he had never walked a picket line – observers noted that his own record of achievement was not overly impressive. If AFL–CIO membership had fallen by a fifth since the merger, UAW membership had declined by a similar amount, prompting jibes from his enemies that he should be looking to his own patch. Like other unions, the UAW was beginning to lose representation ballots which previously might have been won, and a long-planned recruitment drive among white-collar workers produced no dramatic results. A. H. Raskin argued that Reuther had no better formula for organising the unorganised than Meany, and pointed out that the IUD under Reuther's leadership had a staff jaded by seven years of loud talk and little action.[20] A friendly observer, John Herling, agreed that Reuther needed to work at revitalising the labour movement and restoring the credibility of the industrial unions: 'it is not enough,' he wrote, 'to talk, as Walter Reuther frequently does, about "little men of little vision", without showing exactly how men increase in stature and improve their outlook. This is what Mr Reuther's durable friends and dour critics both are saying. Outside of his own considerable union, is Mr Reuther just a gymnasium fighter?'[21]

A major part of the problem was that affluence was making it hard to recapture the spirit of the 1930s, a fact that Reuther was all too well aware of. As he told the 1962 UAW convention: 'A labor movement can get soft and flabby spiritually. It can make progress materially and the soul of the union can die in the process.'[22] Colleagues had been advising him of the need for labour to mend its fences with the liberal intellectual community which had lost faith in the movement, believing that the trade unions had no philosophy, no ideology. Others urged an active policy for the UAW regarding the dispossessed, migrant labour and minorities. Such people were in danger of becoming alienated from the labour movement because of the way they were exploited and ignored. Tackling their problems would create a climate conducive to more organising success and lessen the danger of further anti-union legislation.[23]

Reuther's response in this situation was to immerse himself in a series of major domestic and international initiatives, working through the UAW, the IUD and the IMF, while soft-pedalling his relations with Meany and the AFL–CIO in an attempt to establish a *détente* in that organisation. At home in early 1963, alongside his civil rights activities, he launched a major $4 million organising initiative by the IUD in key cities, targeting specific industries and firms. Overall direction of the IUD was handed over to Reuther's close ally Jack Conway, and his brother Roy was drafted in to assist with the programme.

However, Reuther conceived of labour's interests not merely in national terms, and with new hands on the levers of foreign policy in the early 1960s, there was scope for constructive work in asserting labour's values on a wider international scale. He was very clear in his understanding of how the international climate affected trade union fortunes at home, and he seized the opportunity afforded by Kennedy's presidency to forge new political alliances abroad. It was this sort of boldness of initiative and breadth of vision that really distinguished Reuther from his fellow labour leaders.

The growth of 'revisionism' within European Social Democracy from the late 1950s encouraged Reuther to believe that opportunities were opening up for greater co-operation between American progressives and the European left. He had sent Adolph Sturmthal to Europe to report to him on political developments there, and from 1961 a number of parallel initiatives suggested the possibility of creating an international movement that would harness the new political forces on both sides of the Atlantic. In August 1961 Wilhelm Gefeller, leader of the German Chemical Workers' Union, visited Detroit and suggested to Reuther the idea of creating a broad international coalition embracing the ICFTU, the international trade secretariats, the Christian trade unions and the various Christian and Social Democratic parties whose purpose would be to develop a unified political approach to the problems raised by the developing world. Sturmthal had also raised with Reuther the idea of forming an international organisation of American liberals and the non-communist left which he and the White House adviser, Arthur Schlesinger, had been discussing. At the same time the Italian politicians Altiero Spinelli and Ugo La Malfa were proposing the creation of a body to promote in an international setting the sort of political realignment then in prospect in Italy through the 'opening to the left'.[24] In essence these proposals all pointed to the promotion of centre-left coalition politics on a multinational basis.

Out of these independent initiatives an attempt was made to form a transatlantic movement, the International Study Group on Freedom and Democracy, to press for social change through democratic means. The rationale that particularly appealed to Reuther was that there existed no forum in which progressives from across the non-communist world could exchange ideas and discuss policies. The Americans were not members of the Socialist International, which in any case had little authority, and the ICFTU was limited in its range of activities and was greatly handicapped by its conflicts with Meany and his supporters. As Sturmthal and Schlesinger saw it, the need was for an association of progressive and politically influential people to exert pressure within particular countries in the cause of social justice, pushing cautious governments forward while, in the spirit of Kennedy's New Frontier and the Alliance for Progress, the American administration exerted pressure from outside. All this was based on a fashionable belief that the differences between capitalism and social democracy were dissolving. Walter Reuther helped fund the Study Group and Victor was a member of its Advisory Council. With its planned programme of training and education for democracy in various countries, it remained a peripheral organisation, but the thinking behind it which had attracted Reuther was now pursued more directly through the Harpsund conferences.

The Harpsund conferences were a series of informal meetings of world social democratic and labour leaders which Reuther helped organise. They took place annually at Harpsund in Sweden from 1963 to 1965 and were held under the auspices of the Swedish Social Democrats. Reuther was very much the driving force behind the initiative. It grew out of discussions that he had with Willy Brandt in 1962 on the need for closer liaison between the non-doctrinaire left and for more effective contact with the intellectual and political leadership of the emerging nations. Brandt agreed to float the idea before the Swedish Prime Minister, Tage Erlander and the British Labour Party leader, Hugh Gaitskell, and then left it to Reuther to follow up in making the arrangements. Reuther secured Erlander's agreement to host the meeting, and then approached Hubert Humphrey, Senate majority leader, and Arthur Schlesinger to urge American participation.[25]

The first meeting was held at Harpsund over two days in July 1963 and included among the small group of participants Erlander, Brandt, Harold Wilson, Hubert Humphrey, Erich Ollenhauer, and leaders from the German, Swedish and Norwegian trade union centres. They discussed economic integration, expansion and full employment, disarmament and the problems of developing countries. Reuther spoke forcefully of the dangers and opportunities presented by automation, and in the process provided Harold Wilson with material for the 'white hot technological revolution' theme with which he successfully fought the next British general election. As the future Prime Minister wrote to Reuther the following month:

> I regard the Harpsund meeting as one of the very greatest importance – you will have seen that speaking at the Durham Miners Gala the following Saturday, I made the automation and employment problem the main theme of my speech. This attracted a great deal of press attention and comment: the figures I quoted were largely based on the material you gave to me.

Reuther and Humphrey met President Kennedy on their return to report on the conference, while Brandt wrote to Reuther that such talks should be held regularly. [26]

At Reuther's suggestion, the meeting established a study group of economic experts to examine the international monetary arrangements necessary to ease British and American balance of payments difficulties in the context of full employment policy. The reform of the international monetary system became the central concern of the Harpsund meetings, the aim being to devise techniques for strengthening the International Monetary Fund and creating a world monetary system that would foster full employment and healthy economic growth in the industrialised countries, together with rapid development in the emerging nations. There was optimism for reform in this direction following the British Labour Party's election victory in 1964, the creation of a centre-left government in Italy, the fact that the United States administration had recently adopted a more open-minded approach, and with the looming possibility of a Brandt-led SPD government in Germany. As UAW economist Nat Weinberg remarked to Reuther, if the SPD won the next German election, Harpsund could become the catalyst for promoting a new orthodoxy. [27] This was exactly Reuther's hope.

Consideration was given to widening the membership of the group, but in fact at the follow-up meeting in Harpsund in July–August 1964 the trend was in the opposite direction and Hubert Humphrey was prevented from attending by Lyndon Johnson. Humphrey aspired to be US Vice-President, but as Johnson pointed out, the Harpsund meeting to which he had been invited was a gathering of socialists. [28] Here was a genuine conflict of interests. Reuther's participation at Harpsund was motivated by a desire to overcome the isolation of the American labour and liberal community at not being part of the international socialist fraternity. Much of his international activity was intended to establish a network of allies within the broad labour and socialist movement without having to seek membership of the Socialist International. However, in the United States the word 'socialist' was beyond the bounds of political acceptability, and since the vice-presidency was at stake, Reuther did not demur at Johnson's decision. Indeed, when it was suggested that the report of the Harpsund working party on international monetary issues be submitted to the Socialist International, Reuther was advised to omit his own name from the document. [29]

Yet a collective belief that a new political age might be about to dawn kept contacts between the Harpsund partners close. Reuther lunched with Prime Minister Harold Wilson, Willy Brandt and leading British trade unionists at Downing Street in November 1964, after which Brandt wrote to Reuther urging the need to find a way of bringing Humphrey back into the circle: 'It is important to keep up the Harpsund contact and it would be ideal if Harold would arrange for a meeting in which Hubert could participate.'[30] Three weeks later, with Wilson in Washington for a meeting with Johnson, Reuther was hospitalised and was forced to miss a scheduled dinner with the two leaders (he was operated on for a growth on his lung), but he wrote to tell the British Prime Minister that he would be in touch with the President and Humphrey while in hospital and would intervene if Wilson thought he could help. It was particularly important for Wilson to impress on Johnson and Humphrey continued participation in Harpsund.[31] In the event, Johnson did agree to Humphrey's attendance at the third Harpsund gathering in 1965, and the Vice-President was only prevented from going by the pressure of domestic politics.

While the Harpsund programme aimed to cement ties between centre-left governments, the most spectacular instance of such politics in the making was in Italy in the early 1960s, and there Reuther also played an important part. In Italy, the notion of a political 'opening to the left' had long been discussed, but during the Eisenhower years the Americans were unwilling to lend their support. Now, with Kennedy as President, American government policy encouraged moves to bring the Italian Socialists and Social Democrats into a coalition with the Christian Democrats. A key element in transforming the political balance was the strengthening of the position of socialists within the trade union movement. As Reuther observed, the new coalition would remain precarious until the political alliance found expression in trade union ranks.[32] He performed an important role in bringing this about, aiming in practice to reinforce the position of Nenni Socialists and Saragat Social Democrats, and restricting the capacity of communist trade unionists to sabotage the evolving political settlement.

Working closely with the Kennedy administration, his initial role was to encourage the belief among the Italian leaders that a new political order was now imperative. The State Department and the American Embassy in Rome were still not fully behind Kennedy's policy, and the Italians needed to be convinced of the Americans' true position. In

May 1961, therefore, Reuther held talks in Rome with Nenni, Saragat and the Christian Democrat Prime Minister Amintore Fanfani to urge the change. Back in the United States, he met Robert Kennedy at his home and then attended a session of the National Security Council where he urged the need for American officials in Italy to be given a new brief.[33] The upshot of this diplomacy was that in February 1962 Saragat's Social Democrats entered a Christian Democrat-led coalition, with Nenni's support, though without his participation – the 'partial turn to the left'. Further diplomatic efforts were directed at Nenni, while Reuther met with administration staff to report on the lack of sympathy for the new policy on the part of the US labour attaché in Rome, and to press for his replacement.[34]

In June 1962 he was again in Italy for talks with Nenni and several trade union leaders, this time to arrange for the financing of the socialist trade unionists. In 1962 the UAW and the metalworkers' unions of Germany, Sweden, Austria and Switzerland established the International Labor Education Fund in a 'discreet effort to assist the consolidation of Italian democratic unionism'. The fund was separate from the IMF, but the Federation's general secretary, Adolph Graedel, acted as treasurer and the fund was based in his private residence. The money was used for 'several large-scale educational programmes' that continued until 1966. Apart from this, there was also a second fund subscribed to jointly by the UAW and the American Amalgamated Clothing Workers (ACW) intended specifically for use by the Nenni group in the Italian Socialist Party (PSI).[35]

American attention was focused on the general election in April 1963, out of which it was hoped to bring the Nenni Socialists into the coalition – the 'full opening to the left'. With this in mind Reuther returned to Italy again in March 1963 for meetings with Nenni, Saragat and Fanfani and returned optimistic about the election outcome. The election result was inconclusive, and immediate participation in government by the Nenni group was prevented by a split in his party. Further progress had to await the outcome of the PSI congress in October where Nenni needed to secure a majority for his policy. Fabio Cavazza, secretary of the European wing of the International Study Group on Freedom and Democracy, wrote to tell Reuther that for Nenni to triumph at the congress he would need to exercise tight control of the delegates by influencing the outcomes of the 100 or so prior provincial party congresses, and that the cost of organising this support would be some $90,000.[36] To assist Nenni's struggle within the party, Reuther dispatched $16,377 to Italy in the summer of 1963, matching a similar amount from the ACW. This financing helped Nenni's campaign to commit the party to the coalition. By the end of the year they were full partners in a centre-left government, Nenni as deputy prime minister and Saragat as foreign minister, and in a position to tackle the economic and social welfare reforms long overdue in Italy.

For a time, the demagogic militancy of the communist trade union-ists was the biggest threat to the new settlement, and the need to strengthen the non-communist wing took on a new urgency. In November 1965 Reuther was asked to find within the United States a further $40,000 for training socialist union activists in Italy. Shortly afterwards, when a plan for the mass defection of socialist members from the communist-led trade union centre was under consideration, Reuther was informed that, as a matter of urgency, American labour sympathisers would need to contribute half a million Swiss francs out of a total $1\frac{1}{2}$ million to ensure that the breakaway group still had organisational resources.[37] In the event, the break did not take place and what, if any, direct assistance Reuther gave on this occasion is unclear. However, on the advice of Hubert Humphrey's staff, Victor Reuther did suggest to Walter that he should see President Johnson directly on the issue: 'If the President gives the green light then we can set up the other meetings to discuss specifics and details.'[38]

In 1963, the year that the Harpsund meetings began, Reuther stepped up his activities in the international trade union movement. The pre-vious year the UAW had created the International Free World Labor Defense Fund financed from the interest deriving from the UAW's strike fund. Initially, with the strike fund standing at $25 million, it was to yield an annual income of $1.5 million to assist with labour projects overseas, and the strike fund itself later grew to over $40 million. There were numerous beneficiaries of this fund, the earlier ones including French miners, who received $25,000 in the course of an early strike against de Gaulle's arbitrary exercise of power; Italian socialist trade union members; the underground union coalition in Spain, which was building a network of support in preparation for the collapse of the Franco regime; metalworkers in Turkey, whose union was largely built with UAW assistance; Kenneth Kaunda's United

National Independence party, then about to contest the first free elections in Zambia; and Michael Manley, at the time a Jamaican trade union leader, whose legal costs in a labour court case were covered by Reuther.

However, Reuther was not engaged in random philanthropy, and the bulk of UAW effort and expenditure in this new phase of international activity was devoted to systematic programmes within the IMF that he saw as important for the well-being of American autoworkers. It was perhaps his most imaginative project as UAW president and was prompted by the growing internationalisation of the automobile industry.

From the mid–1950s, at Reuther's urging, the IMF had been striving to create structures under which workers of particular multinational corporations would maintain close contact. The idea was formally adopted in 1956 with a proposal to create liaison committees for unions representing Ford and GM workers. But progress in turning this simple idea into a working reality was slow. Apart from the general logistical difficulties of sustaining activity such as this internationally, Reuther's strategy aroused principled opposition among some European union leaders, particularly the Germans and British. They feared that the programme would lead to an emphasis on company-level collective bargaining as distinct from the national/industry-level bargaining common in Europe. Mainstream union leaders were worried about the disruption of traditional practices which could jeopardise wider union solidarity, while communist critics accused Reuther of promoting corporatist labour–management relations at the level of single firms while selling out the class struggle.

It was a fundamental issue reflecting the different philosophical approaches of the two trade union traditions, and it had loomed in the background of American–European trade union relations from the earliest days of post-war reconstruction in Europe and throughout the Marshall Plan years. The Americans could never accept that effective trade unionism was possible in a situation where collective agreements were made at a distant industry or national level and without reasonable assurance of being policed through a formal system of plant-based representatives and grievance procedures. On this they were convinced they had something to teach the Europeans. Company-level bargaining was the norm in the United States auto industry, and for tactical reasons the UAW had always avoided the prospect of a nationwide dispute, preferring to manoeuvre between the corporations and play one off against another. They maintained that in countries where bargaining was conducted on a national basis, the outcome was determined by the needs of marginal firms, meaning that large multinational corporations were under little pressure to pay what they could afford. Even to organise a union in one country in the face of opposition from the multinational firm was extremely difficult unless the union with which the parent firm dealt was prepared to assist by exerting pressure at the nerve centre. The UAW were sensitive to the European fears about this and tried to reassure them that it was not the intention to substitute some novel approach to collective bargaining,[39] yet this was the ultimate logic of the strategy.

To win support for the project, Reuther dispatched Victor to Britain to meet Transport and General Workers' Union (T&GWU) leader Frank Cousins, while he himself went to Germany and spoke at an IG Metall conference of autoworkers in Bremen in 1958. Constantly in his mind was the international wage differential: American autoworkers earned almost four times the wages of German workers and two-and-a-half times the Swedish wage, while the Swedes earned three times the Japanese wage, and all were working with roughly the same kind of technology. It allowed American employers to sideswipe the UAW, as when the chairman of Ford later praised European unions for their contribution to economic stability: 'No small contribution has been made by the wise and statesmanlike union leaders and workers in England, Germany and other countries, who repeatedly refused to press for wage increases because they felt their country could not afford them.'[40]

The link between such differentials and protectionist sentiment in the USA was obvious, and Reuther stressed in Bremen that the more Germans were able to raise their wages, the easier it would be for American labour to resist the calls for raising tariff barriers. Pointing to the size of German car exports and the lack of car ownership in Germany, he argued that no nation could be permanently prosperous simply by relying on the export trade: it needed also a strong domestic market based on high wages. But with only 30 per cent of Volkswagen workers unionised, Ford of Germany less than 15 per cent unionised, and with no direct wage negotiations between the firm and the union, he accused the German auto industry of 'wage dumping'.

The problem of international wage differentials began to be particu-

larly serious in 1959 as the threat of foreign competition from countries with lower labour costs increased, and as the trend for American
firms to relocate abroad grew. American corporations claimed that
high wages made them uncompetitive, suggesting the need to erect
tariff barriers, relocate production overseas, or attack high wages in
America. All these options were unacceptable to Reuther, for whom
the real alternative was to focus on ways of raising wages in competitor
countries. His solution was based on the concept of unfair labour
standards which would be deemed to exist, and would be a target for
union action, where remuneration was less than productivity allowed:
in other words, where unit labour costs were significantly lower than
in the importing country.[41]

The UAW argued its case within the IMF at a protracted series of
meetings between 1959 and 1961. The aim was to secure agreement
on a policy under which international fair labour standards, so defined,
would be urged as a feature of international trade agreements under
GATT. The proposal aroused considerable controversy in the IMF,
with some European members objecting that it was playing into the
employers' hands to accept the link between wages and productivity;
that it was folly to rely on intergovernmental regulation of fair wages
rather than traditional collective bargaining methods, and arguing anyway that less developed countries should be allowed to take advantage
of their cheap labour costs in order to benefit more generally from the
industrialisation that would follow. The IMF was not wholly convinced
of the merits of Reuther's approach, and not until 1971 did the Federation accept, even in a diluted form, the idea of intergovernmental
intervention.

However, the spotlight now firmly shone on the problem caused by
international wage competition, and Reuther attempted to tackle directly what would become the main threat to American automobile
workers – low-cost imports from Japan. His activities here closely
paralleled his work in Italy. Winning the ideological battle against
communism within Japanese labour was an initial aim, but unlike
George Meany, who was also vitally concerned with Japanese developments, he was determined to support the more militant elements in
the Japanese movement. By 1960 it was in danger of splitting between
an eastern form of business unionism and a communist-inspired wing
given to revolutionary rhetoric and political mobilisation, but unable
to deliver gains at the workplace or in the economic field. In practice,

Reuther's strategy involved encouraging the non-communist leadership that was beginning to emerge in Sohyo, the largest union centre, and promoting unity between it and its smaller and more moderate rival Zenro (later named Domei). In metalworking industries, it meant building up a Japanese section of the IMF in order to overcome the fragmentation of the enterprise unions. Japanese auto unionism was weak, with separate enterprise unions at Toyota, Isuzu, Hino and Nissan, only the latter having any success in organising the many workers employed by subcontractors. As ever, it was Reuther's view that the best way of defeating communism and serving the interests of union members was to build a democratic movement that was capable of industrial militancy. However, in this case the promotion of militant wage bargaining in Japan was also meant to serve directly the cause of American labour.

A series of reciprocal visits by UAW and Japanese auto union members began, and in 1962 Reuther himself went to Japan in his multiple capacity as leader of the ICFTU, IMF and UAW. He wanted the visit to be a catalyst for labour unity in the country, and much diplomatic effort was made to ensure that his invitation was extended by all the competing labour centres. During a two-week stay in November 1962, he worked to bring the mutually suspicious leaders together, and his efforts culminated in a joint statement issued at the end of the visit which envisaged the creation of a wage research centre embracing all sections of the Japanese labour movement.[42]

The idea was his and was intended to promote Japanese labour unity by forcing the rival groups to work together, while providing a mechanism for highlighting the low wages in Japan. It also aimed to draw the Japanese further into the international labour fraternity since the bulk of the finances for the centre were to be from American and European sources, with significant contributions from the ICFTU and the IMF. It was important that the centre be seen to be an international operation if its statistical output were to have any credibility, since Japanese official figures were inclined to be suspect. It was Reuther's view that the availability of reliable statistical information about the level and composition of labour remuneration in Japan would facilitate a different style of trade unionism with an emphasis on militant collective bargaining based on wage comparisons, rather than, as in the past, an enterprise-oriented concern for increasing productivity and pay geared to what employers claimed they could afford. Yet he also believed that a full costing of wages and fringe benefits would show the differential with other countries to be less than often imagined, and this would help the anti-protectionist cause, of which he was a devout supporter.

However, the value of the joint statement was soon called into question as the conservative Zenro leadership began to back-track, clearly fearful that the result of any wage survey might be severely embarrassing to them. Aware that George Meany had no sympathy for what Reuther was attempting, they questioned whether he had actually been speaking for the AFL–CIO. Although Reuther sent $25,000 to Japan before the end of 1963 as part of a joint UAW–IUD commitment to cover a third of the centre's annual operating costs, the AFLC–IO itself declined to be directly involved in the venture. Progress in launching the research centre was therefore slow and it was not until autumn 1965, nearly three years after his visit, that the new organisation actually began work. By early 1968, comparative international studies had been completed of wage costs in four industries including automobiles, but then Domei (formerly Zenro) indicated that it was withdrawing support for the activity.[43]

The fact was that mutual suspicions among the various Japanese centres increased during the 1960s rather than disappearing in the wake of this collaborative effort. In part it was the success of Reuther's strategy of pressing for closer federation on the part of the metal-working unions that contributed to the failure of the wider policy of promoting labour unity. In 1964 the IMF launched a Japanese Council (IMF–JC) bringing together various metalworking unions. Whereas initially it was intended as a bridge between Sohyo and Zenro/Domei, attracting affiliations from unions belonging to each organisation, increasingly it came to be seen as a rival body. At the same time it pursued a moderate industrial programme that reflected the conservative values of the Meany-backed Zenro/Domei. Reuther's strategy for militant collective bargaining hinged on an ability to build on the more vigorous, democratic elements of Sohyo, but the emergence of the IMF–JC was to mark the beginning of a long-term erosion of that centre's position in the private sector.

The difficulty of constructing a practical policy around the concept of international fair labour standards increased the need for unions to be more cohesive in their direct dealings with employers. Promoting co-ordination across borders was a laborious process with no likelihood of early rewards, but Reuther kept up the pressure for international co-operation. In his presidential address to the IMF's automotive conference in November 1960 he called on all affiliated unions to notify the Federation of the schedule of their negotiations, and urged sister organisations to supply whatever data was necessary to strengthen the presentation of their case in negotiations. By way of injecting the UAW more directly into their collective bargaining, he proposed that affiliated unions based in the home country of the corporations be asked to provide a staff adviser to work with the national union bargaining representatives. He promoted international exchange visits of workplace leaders, aimed at bringing home to workers of different nationalities the fact that they really were employed by the same corporation. To this end, eighty-two local UAW leaders from Detroit visited Europe in 1960 alone. 'It is now very urgent,' Reuther wrote, 'that our secondary leadership from first hand knowledge discover that our automobile economy is now dominated by *international* companies. The sooner they understand this the more likely it is we will be able to begin to plan an effective strategy for this new era.'[44] Slowly, concrete signs of co-operation began to appear, the German metalworkers collaborating with the UAW in the organisation of workers in the new Volkswagen plant in Canada, and with the UAW involved in a major effort to unionise the Ford plant at Cologne in the early 1960s.

However, when Reuther stressed the need for the IMF to devote more of its resources to campaigns in particular industries such as auto manufacture, rather than for general organising activities in metalworking, he met fierce resistance from the German metalworkers' leadership. Subsequent arguments between them about centralised versus decentralised structures in the IMF were essentially arguments about the whole Reuther strategy. In 1964 he pressed for the liaison committees – now termed world co-ordinating councils – to be extended to cover workers at Chrysler, Fiat and Volkswagen, together with the creation of a more effective information and co-ordinating centre for auto unions. The Federation's German president, Otto Brenner, prevaricated, and at an executive committee meeting in Vienna in November 1964 the UAW came close to threatening to leave the organisation if the programme were held back. However, as the largest single contributor to the IMF's coffers, with $250,000 earmarked for its solidarity fund in 1964 alone, Reuther was in a position to insist on having his way.

He followed this up in 1965 by securing IMF agreement to appoint a UAW official, Herman Rebhan, as auto co-ordinator for the IMF, with his salary paid by the UAW and initially based in the UAW head office in Detroit. Driving the policy hard, Reuther convened meetings of the world co-ordinating councils in Detroit in June 1966 where, for the first time, they adopted a common commitment to specific collective bargaining goals in what was hailed as the Declaration of Detroit. The programme involved pursuit of common improvements in hours, premium payments, security of employment, retirement age and pensions, union rights and grievance procedures. The IMF embarked on an international comparison of jobs and wages in the industry and was now capable of exchanging considerably more information on collective bargaining provisions, obviating the chances of sub-standard agreements being negotiated through ignorance. An organisational programme to extend the coverage of the world councils to Latin America began, and the Federation assisted with collective bargaining activities of autoworkers from Australia to Venezuela and Mexico, where Reuther had recently been to help found a Mexican Autoworkers' Council.

It was well understood that the prospect of co-ordinated collective bargaining on an international basis was a long way off. However, without raising members' expectations too high, Reuther believed that it was realistic to press for standardisation of some economic benefits within common trading blocs such as the EEC where the goals of a forty-hour week and upward wage harmonisation were now adopted as bargaining targets. Common global aims were restricted to non-economic matters where Reuther hoped for dramatic improvements. He envisaged the next stage of the strategy involving working towards common expiry dates of agreements and the identification of target plants in each region as a focal point of upwardly-harmonising campaigns, or even for a concerted effort to increase membership and strengthen in-plant union structures.

The entire programme in the automobile industry was attributable to Reuther's efforts. It was practical trade unionism applied in an international setting, making a daily reality of the concept of international brotherhood that most other union leaders reserved only for Sunday speeches. Tangible gains were beginning to be made as bargaining lessons were transmitted from one country to another: the late 1960s and early 70s were a high watermark of hopes for international trade unionism. Shortcomings in the programme reflected deficiencies in national labour movements beyond his control. The limitations of the Japanese unions held back the creation of world co-ordinating councils at Nissan and Toyota. The lack of any co-ordinating structure at British Leyland reflected the traditional insularity of the British unions, rarely more than spectators in IMF affairs until, on Reuther's initiative, Jack Jones of the Transport and General Workers' Union and Hugh Scanlon of the Amalgamated Engineering Union agreed with him to convene a series of annual tripartite seminars for the leaders of their three unions beginning in 1969.

Ultimately the programme required more internationalisation of union structures which required national unions surrendering some of their autonomy. With its enhanced programme of international co-operation agreed in 1966, the IMF could congratulate itself on its foresight. But worldwide corporate rationalisation in the automobile industry that followed in the next five years suggested that unions would shortly face an environment even more hostile than hitherto envisaged. As Reuther wrote in the British labour weekly, *Tribune*, in June 1969, less than a year before his death:

> there is no room left for purely national trade unionism. Even less is there room for what might be called trade union colonialism. In the decade of the seventies labor internationally must create and perfect organizational machinery which is responsive to the democratic will of all participants, under the control of no single trade union center or bloc of such centers, and serving the interests of workers everywhere, irrespective of national boundaries or possibly conflicting national interests.

The IMF, with its world co-ordinating councils, was clearly his preferred model, and that vision of practical international trade unionism was his legacy to the labour movement.[45]

Reuther's shift of attention in 1962 from domestic AFL–CIO politics to the labour movement's wider social and international interests ushered in a period of apparent harmony in the Federation. He exercised self-restraint in his dealings with Meany, but his distaste at the way the AFL–CIO was being administered was undiminished and he began to keep a record of personal slights and failures of leadership by the AFL–CIO president. The relative tranquility in AFL–CIO affairs was finally shattered in May 1966 when Victor Reuther gave an interview to the *Los Angeles Times* in which he denounced the CIA financing of American labour activities overseas. Press reports of the labour movement's contacts with American intelligence had begun to appear in 1965, and in a steady stream the details were coming into the public domain. Lovestoneism had never been stamped out: indeed, Lovestone's formal standing had been enhanced in 1964 when he was made director of the AFL–CIO International Affairs Department, thus confirming what had previously been *de facto* his responsibility for international policy. Moreover, the formation of AIFLD in 1961, followed in 1964 by a parallel organisation for channelling aid to Africa, the African–American Labor Center (AALC), had increased significantly the scope for intelligence agency operations within the labour field.

As the UAW's international director, Victor Reuther monitored closely these developments. He had continuously pressed his brother to challenge Meany over Lovestone's role, and his statement to the press in May 1966 was thought by some to be motivated by a desire to force a confrontation on the matter. Certainly, Walter Reuther was angered by Victor's disclosure and told Meany that the statement should never have been made. However, international events now developed a momentum of their own, and within days of Victor's statement, Meany and Reuther were at loggerheads over the withdrawal of the AFL–CIO delegation at the International Labour Organisation (ILO) Conference following the election of a Polish communist delegate to the presidency. This Cold War gesture had not been sanctioned by the AFL–CIO executive committee and Reuther protested vigorously at Meany's support for it.[46]

The fact of the CIA financing of labour activities was scheduled to be discussed at the AFL–CIO executive council in August 1966, but strenuous efforts were made by the administration to kill public discussion of the issue. Vice-President Hubert Humphrey and Senator Robert Kennedy both called Reuther and asked him not to force debate on the matter. Reuther was agreeable but was not prepared to initiate steps to have the issue withdrawn. Only when Meany also declared his willingness to remove the CIA connection from the agenda did he concur. However, when the executive council meeting convened, the issue of Victor Reuther's allegation found its way on to the agenda. Walter Reuther believed that he had been ambushed and that it was no longer possible to trust Meany's word. His assistant, Jack

Conway, who had mediated between the two men over the executive council agenda, believed that this was the final straw as far as the UAW president was concerned.[47]

The indications are that Reuther was bounced into a position of open conflict with Meany by his brother's action. He had been reluctant to engage in hostilities with Meany on this issue: the initial rebuke to Victor and his willingness to accede to administration requests to avoid public discussion of the matter were testimony to this. Yet now that the facts were in the open Reuther was carried along on an irresistible tide of opposition to almost all that Meany stood for, a tide that led inexorably to the UAW quitting the AFL–CIO, and its president being isolated from the rest of the labour movement.

In the decade that began with the high hopes of the New Frontier and then sank into the mire of the Vietnam War, Reuther experienced mixed fortunes. With ready access to two Presidents, he was at the peak of his power, a leading figure among those urging a firmer commitment to the goals of the Great Society. Yet administration performance never matched the promise of its early rhetoric. Reuther's strategy since the 1950s had been to manoeuvre himself into a position where he could influence Democratic Party policies in ways beneficial to labour, but the experience of the 1960s raised questions about the usefulness of that approach. Nonetheless, he was one of the most important white figures behind the successes of the civil rights movement and a powerful driving force in the extensive anti-poverty programmes of the decade. In collective bargaining, Reuther continued to set the pace for the rest of organised labour, widening the range of negotiated fringe benefits that workers would later come to expect as of right. The affluent mid–sixties were a period in which the auto employers could well afford these concessions, but nothing was ever given away, and the UAW gains, as in 1964, were won only through lengthy industrial action.

Reuther's most striking achievements, though, were in the international field, where he demonstrated a breadth of vision unique in the labour movement, working hard for political and social change, both for the benefits it would bestow on workers abroad and as a way of protecting the interests of his members at home. The growing hopes for international union co-operation in collective bargaining that blossomed in the late 1960s were very much the result of his pioneering work. Yet at the back of all this Reuther had to contend with a deteriorating situation within the AFL–CIO, always conservative and bureaucratic, and in international matters increasingly reactionary. He had studiously avoided open conflict with George Meany up to the mid–sixties, despite a growing disenchantment with his leadership. At length the public rupture came in 1966 with Reuther's willingness to trust Meany finally exhausted. It had been his ambition to succeed to the AFL–CIO presidency, but the course he was now embarked on would soon see him outside the mainstream of the American trade union movement and waging a lonely campaign for labour's soul.

7 The last years

The Vietnam War was the dominant factor in American life in the late 1960s. It polarised society and undermined scope for the social reform at home to which Reuther was committed. It also provided the backdrop for his last years as UAW president, and yet on the issue of the war he was regarded as no more than a moderate dove.[1] In truth he was unwilling to give up the prospect of political influence by criticising the President, and he was prepared to be conciliatory within the hawkish AFL–CIO in order to achieve a uniform labour policy. When his brother Victor expressed public disapproval of the war, Reuther lambasted him: 'What the hell are you doing, you YPSL, annoying Johnson like that? You know that isn't UAW policy.'[2] (The YPSL – 'yipsils' – were the Young People's Socialist League to which the brothers had belonged in the 1930s. By calling him a yipsil, Reuther was telling him he was undisciplined.)

It was ironic that the foremost labour proponent of disarmament should have become a tacit defender of this military venture long after large sections of America turned against it. Like many others, he agonised over the war, but remained loyal to President Johnson while advocating the UAW line in favour of a politically negotiated settlement. With many union members and sons of members in Vietnam, he refused to say that their sacrifices were futile, even as domestic spending on social and anti-poverty programmes began to be cut as a result of military expenditure. When Johnson finally terminated the bombing of North Vietnam, Reuther wrote to him applauding his courageous act of statesmanship and assuring him of the autoworkers' unwavering support.[3] By 1969 he was among those advocating peace talks in Paris, coupled with an immediate ceasefire. But he resisted the advice of some of his union colleagues that he should dissociate himself from the war, and he refused to sign a statement calling for a unilateral withdrawal from Vietnam.

Reuther's position had been close to that of Robert Kennedy in

1968, and some maintain that he might have supported the New York Senator's candidacy for President. As it was, he threw his weight behind his old ally Hubert Humphrey while strongly urging the Vice-President to distance himself from Johnson's policies. Reuther actually drafted a campaign speech along these lines for Humphrey and flew to his Minnesota home in the hope of persuading him to use it. Humphrey seemed agreeable, but the speech was never delivered and he went into the 1968 presidential election totally identified with Johnson's Vietnam policy.[4] Reuther had compromised a great deal in order to remain on the right side of the Democratic establishment, but once the cost of war began to eat into the Great Society programmes, the gains from this strategy were increasingly illusory. The UAW leadership became disillusioned by the experience, aware that labour had been largely taken for granted by the Democrats.

Reuther's support for the Johnson/Humphrey line on Vietnam enraged students, and he was heckled at meetings of Students for a Democratic Society (SDS), despite being one of their benefactors. One of his self-justifications – that it was an inappropriate time to break with the President because of the approach of major collective bargaining – cut no ice with idealistic youth, and his own college-age daughter later wrote that she came to see him as part of the problem.[5] It was only days before his death in May 1970, following the American bombing of Cambodia and the killing of students at Kent State University that Reuther, in his last message as UAW president, declared that 'the highest form of patriotism and human morality is to insist that America end the tragic war and loss of life'.[6]

Despite his stand on the war, which caused disillusionment among many liberals, his long-term commitment had been to a reduction in the military budget. He had argued for years that the only war worth fighting was the war against poverty, and since the early 1960s he had trumpeted the cause of arms conversion. The UAW urged the appointment of a Commission on the Economics of Disarmament, whose purpose would be to prepare new programmes to ease the impact of disarmament on particular communities as a result of arms conversion. In December 1969 Reuther testified before the Senate Labor and Public Welfare Committee in favour of a requirement that arms producers put aside a portion of their profits as a 'conversion reserve'.[7] Many of his ideas on this subject were contained in Senator George McGovern's National Economic Conversion Bill of 1969 which gave particular encouragement to the process of conversion for socially useful ends, such as low-cost housing, educational and health facilities and anti-pollution devices. For this, SANE proposed to award him the Eleanor Roosevelt Peace Award, despite his refusal to advocate their policy of a unilateral withdrawal from Vietnam.

At home the economic and social strains generated by the Vietnam war were felt by the union in the form of a growing rank-and-file revolt – of skilled workers, who had seen the value of their wages eroded, of disaffected young workers out of tune with their leadership, and of black workers influenced by the growing militancy of the black power movement and suffering from the cutbacks in the Great Society programmes. Reuther had supported Martin Luther King, Philip Randolph and the established black leadership, but he was out of sympathy with the new generation of militant black activists in Detroit, and they were among the keenest opponents of his leadership in the late sixties.

In the early years of the decade, dissident blacks in the auto union were already working autonomously, supporting their preferred mayoral candidate in Detroit against the UAW-endorsed candidate. Later, the formation within the UAW of the black Dodge Revolutionary Union Movement (DRUM), with its violent language of Third World liberation movements, marked a significant escalation in the militancy of black workers. Following the 1967 Detroit riots, Reuther lobbied with Henry Ford and the President of General Motors for the passing of fair housing legislation. However, he was now on the wrong side of many black leaders in Detroit, who felt he was out of touch and did not understand their problems. He had marched with blacks at Jackson and Selma, answering a personal request from Martin Luther King to do so after demonstrators had been roughly handled by state troopers. He had been present in Charleston supporting a strike of 300 black women, and was the only member of the AFL–CIO executive council to join with the garbage strikers in Memphis at the time of King's assassination. Yet critics claimed that such activities were his way of campaigning for black votes where it was safe. They contrasted the vigour with which the UAW disciplined workers who broke the no-strike pledge, with the moderation with which they treated workers guilty of racial discrimination.[8] 'Reuther,' claimed one opponent, 'is always glad to integrate anything – outside of his own union.'[9]

With the cost of living accelerating as a result of the war in South-East Asia, Reuther approached the 1967 round of bargaining in the knowledge that a significant increase in pay for his skilled members was necessary to restore their confidence in the leadership. He was compelled to adopt an aggressive bargaining stance and, uniquely, to give the skilled trades a veto over any proposed settlement. Profit-sharing was still a favourite theme of the leadership, but there was no likelihood of the corporations accepting it. The union's main objective was salary status for blue-collar workers and the right to strike during the life of an agreement over the growing practice of sub-contracting work. Ironically, an unauthorised strike over this latter issue at a GM plant in Mansfield, Ohio had recently been terminated by the UAW headquarters, and the local union placed under trusteeship. True to Reuther's approach, such unofficial action would not be allowed to interfere with the course of national negotiations, whatever the cause.[10] Successful bargaining, Reuther would tell the membership, 'requires central direction in terms of timing and strategy and tactics, and if we dilute this central direction that is built around authorisation of strikes . . . you dissipate the power of the union at the bargaining table.'[11]

The pattern of settlement in 1967 was established at Ford following a seven-week strike. There were substantial increases in basic pay, especially for skilled workers, and wage parity between US and Canadian autoworkers, seen at the time as a pointer to the future of international collective bargaining. Improved terms in the pension, health insurance and SUB schemes added up to a significant package of economic gains and enabled the union to claim that members and their dependants now enjoyed 'a wide-ranging and substantial defense against the hazards of life extending from cradle to grave'.[12] The basic pattern was applied to GM without strike action, though only after difficult negotiations lasting several months. The heavy price that Reuther had to pay for this was to agree a restriction on the total amount of the wage increase payable under the cost-of-living formula over the coming three years. The cost-of-living 'capping' increased membership discontent, and Reuther would have to reckon with this by the end of the decade.

The 1967 bargaining round was conducted against a background of rapidly deteriorating relations between the UAW and AFL–CIO. This challenged Reuther to demonstrate his effectiveness as a leader, while at the same time, the protracted nature of the negotiations with GM contributed materially to the growing rupture between Reuther and

Meany. Reuther's behaviour within the AFL–CIO was uncharacteristically erratic following his brother's 1966 disclosure of CIA funding of Federation international programmes and the unsuccessful attempt to prevent discussion of this within the executive council. He failed to attend an AFL–CIO executive council meeting in November 1966 that he had requested to discuss international policy. He made sweeping denunciations of the Federation, which were followed in early 1967 by the resignation of UAW officers from their Federation posts. A special UAW convention in April 1967 then adopted a programme of demands for far-reaching reform by the AFL–CIO. However, five days before the Federation convention was due to debate this in December, the UAW announced that, because of the continuing negotiations with GM and the possibility of a strike, its delegates would not be able to attend the convention. Then in March 1968 the UAW demanded that a special AFL–CIO convention be called in December of that year; and when Meany responded by offering to convene it within thirty days provided that the UAW would agree to be bound by its decision, the UAW rejected the offer. The union now refused to pay its affiliation fee, and when its proposal to place this in an escrow account pending resolution of outstanding differences with the Federation was rejected, the UAW was suspended from participation in AFL–CIO affairs in May 1968. The union finally brought the chapter to a close by disaffiliating from the Federation in July 1968.

Altogether, Reuther's tactical handling of this phase of relations with the AFL–CIO lacked finesse. Having attempted over several years to smooth over the tensions within the AFL–CIO while steering it in a more progressive direction, he now seemed to be totally frustrated by his inability to inject more drive and purpose into the organisation and to arouse greater support for his cause among former CIO allies. His differences with Meany ranged across the whole spectrum of labour policy. Indeed, his initial rebuke to Victor Reuther for having exposed the links between the AFL–CIO and the Central Intelligence Agency reflected his view that if there were to be a challenge to Meany's leadership, it would need to be over domestic rather than international issues. The UAW demands for reform of the AFL–CIO were a catalogue of the frustrated hopes that Reuther had entertained since the merger. The labour movement needed to develop an effective political voice; there had to be a substantial increase in the size of union membership, necessitating a big organising drive; the AFL–CIO would have to become a co-ordinator of coalition bargaining, developing effective back-up services and a strong defence fund; and internal reforms would have to be made in the AFL–CIO structure to make it more democratic.

What this might have amounted to in practice was captured in an editorial in the employers' journal, *Factory*:

> Walter Reuther epitomizes the kind of labor leader many managers abhor. He crusades for ideals. He refuses to stage bargaining tangos that mislead his membership. He won't make 'cynical' deals. He exerts every bit of strategic muscle at his command. What's more, he understands – but rarely sympathizes with – managerial economics. All of which makes him a tough, aggressive, thoroughly unpleasant adversary . . . you're not likely to cheer about what may follow if he does get the labor movement going again.[13]

However, with Meany at the helm, reform of the AFL–CIO was out of the question, and though he was well past normal retirement age, he was determined to cling to office and prevent Reuther from succeeding him. For his part, Reuther was now 60 and his capacity for patient waiting was all but exhausted.

According to Frank Winn, a close UAW colleague, the only time Reuther underestimated an adversary was in his judgement of Meany.[14] In this contest, the AFL–CIO president had little difficulty in presenting himself as a long-suffering labour statesman subjected to unwarranted attack by an erratic and jealous opponent. He pointed out that the specific demands now made by Reuther had not been raised during the previous decade; that if he as president was guilty of undemocratic behaviour, the machinery existed for him to be impeached, and if there had been a failure to organise sufficient members in the past it was a failure of the affiliated unions and not just the Federation leadership. Moreover, Meany noted that Reuther himself had been the chairman of the AFL–CIO organising committee for eight years, that he had been largely responsible for appointing its directors, and during that time had only brought in one report which was duly adopted and acted upon. The AFL–CIO account of the dispute was published in a 98-page report, *To Clear the Record*, which curiously Reuther failed to answer.[15]

The UAW's battle with the AFL–CIO reverberated around the international labour movement. In the 1950s ICFTU policy had fuelled the differences between Reuther and Meany, but now the ICFTU became a stage on which they acted out their domestic differences. With the prospect looming of suspension from the AFL–CIO, Reuther wrote to the ICFTU requesting that the UAW be allowed to continue its affiliation to the Confederation as an independent organisation. Days after the UAW's suspension in May 1968 he met ICFTU general secretary, Harm Buiter, in Rome to discuss the possibility. Buiter advised him to apply for renewed membership and indicated that he would support it. For its part the AFL–CIO lobbied hard among ICFTU members to block the move, and in November 1968 the Confederation's executive board voted to take no action on the application. Reuther was stripped of his ICFTU vice-presidency, but the possibility still remained that the UAW might succeed with an appeal against the decision at the Confederation congress in July 1969. Meany was not satisfied that the measures taken to block the UAW were decisive enough and perversely withdrew the AFL–CIO from the ICFTU.

Reuther went ahead with his intention to appeal to the Confederation congress, and Victor Reuther spent many months travelling the world to line up support for their application. Within the UAW there was a feeling that Meany's departure from the world body might prove to be its salvation: the UAW could compensate financially for the loss of AFL–CIO dues, and it might just be possible to restructure the organisation by attracting into membership the more progressive Christian-oriented trade unions, as well as the Czech and Yugoslav trade unions from the liberalising Eastern bloc. However, the prospect of the AFL–CIO detaching itself permanently from the already impoverished ICFTU was more than many key national centres could countenance, and in a bid to woo Meany back into the fold, the British TUC organised a move at the July 1969 congress to keep the UAW application off the agenda. The ploy did not appease the AFL–CIO, but even outside the international body, where it was to remain for over a decade, it was able to exercise an effective veto on Reuther's application for membership. The ICFTU executive board finally rejected the application in December 1969. Reuther was bitter about the lack of support from former CIO colleagues: 'how do you live with people and have any sense of self-respect or any sense of integrity if this is the way you are used,' he complained to his fellow UAW leaders.[16]

For practical purposes, affiliation to the ICFTU was not greatly important, so run-down was the organisation. Still, the UAW had been one of its mainstays, Reuther had had a long association with it and, given his philosophy of the labour movement, it was necessary for him to maintain a prominent role in international affairs. Consequently, more than ever he attached importance to UAW work within the IMF. In line with the growing practice of several European trade union centres – though not the AFL–CIO – he also sought to build bridges to Eastern European labour organisations, capitalising on the emerging climate of détente.

Links were cultivated with the Yugoslav trade union federation. A UAW delegation led by Victor Reuther visited Czechoslovakia and the USSR in the weeks preceding the Soviet invasion of Prague in 1968 and pleaded with Soviet trade union leader Alexander Shelyepin for further liberalisation. For some months after the invasion, the UAW kept up an attempt to liaise with the Czech metalworkers' union, which remained opposed to the new regime. High-level exchange visits with the Romanian metalworkers' union took place, contacts with Polish trade unions were established, and in December 1968 Reuther himself visited Yugoslavia and held talks with President Tito. With the door of the ICFTU closing against him, he was anxious to promote trade union programmes in the Third World and hoped to organise this on a tripartite basis in partnership with the Yugoslavs and the Swedish trade unions, led by his old ally, Arne Geijer.[17]

However, the most remarkable aspect of Reuther's activity following the UAW departure from the AFL–CIO was his attempt to create a new labour centre in the United States based on the UAW and the Teamsters. This was an improbable partnership and certainly reflected the desperation that afflicted Reuther. The Teamsters union had been expelled from the AFL–CIO for the corrupt practices of its leadership, Reuther foremost among its opponents. However, now its president, Jimmy Hoffa, was in prison; a cleaner image was presented to the world, and this, the largest American trade union, had a dynamism that was singularly lacking in most other sections of the labour movement, though its credentials as a socially concerned union were of the flimsiest. Yet together with the Teamsters, Reuther brought the Alliance for Labour Action (ALA) into existence at a convention in May 1969. Its formal structure was sketchy, and publicly Reuther denied that it was meant as a rival centre to the AFL–CIO, though that was the intention if he had been able to attract other unions into membership. In the event, only the Chemical Workers' Union joined with the founding bodies in the ALA. In practice it was little more than a loose alliance for cooperation in specific organising campaigns, for the most part promoting 'community unions'. In 1967 Reuther had described these:

A new concept of union organization has been developing in areas such as Delano and Watts, California. Properly nurtured and motivated, it can spread across the face of the nation, changing the social character of the inner city structure and uplifting the lives of millions of slum dwellers. This new organizing effort is 'the community union'. It is designed to provide the poor with their own self-sufficient economic organization . . . and cuts across many areas of social and economic need . . . health care, schools, public transportation, sanitation, building maintenance etc.[18]

The ALA focused particularly on this kind of self-help organisation and in the process built on existing activities being conducted through the Social, Technical and Educational Programme (STEP). This was a UAW program for collecting supplies and equipment for use in medical, social or educational work in developing countries and deprived parts of the United States. UAW members repaired X-ray machines and other second-hand equipment in their free time, and during the first year of the programme the union transferred $1 million worth of such equipment overseas, providing mobile hospitals and clinics in India, Chile, Brazil and Lebanon, as well as in rural areas of the southern states of the USA. In developing this sort of activity, in conjunction with the ALA's community unions, the UAW now began to draw on the resources of the Free World Labor Defense Fund for projects at home. In this way the Alliance accomplished a good deal in community terms, doing things that most people believed the Teamsters incapable of. Yet its foundation on an unreformed Teamster union was inevitably weak, and it rapidly fell into disuse after Reuther's death. Hardly anyone in the UAW leadership would later defend the ALA, though no-one at the time opposed it. Again, it was a reflection of Reuther's unquestioned dominance as leader of the autoworkers.[19]

His last participation in collective bargaining was in preparation for the 1970 round of negotiations with GM. He had been held responsible by the rank and file for the 1967 agreement which imposed a ceiling on the cost-of-living formula and caused a significant loss in take-home pay. Shop-floor unrest over working conditions arising from the introduction of new technology, contracting out, the ever-present issue of speed-up, and unhealthy working conditions was also reflected in rising absenteeism, an increase in local strikes and a lack of loyalty to the leadership, especially among many younger workers. Aware of this, Reuther conceded:

the speed of production and inspection is too fast: a hundred cars per hour, the required production figure, is too fast for safety and quality. The relation of the human being to the production process is forgotten; the man on the assembly line hasn't got enough time to put six nuts or bolts on before the next block is in front of him.[20]

Like union leaders in Europe who were also faced with an increasingly restive membership, Reuther was conscious that a major shift was taking place in rank-and-file attitudes, but he was unsure of how to handle this situation. His immediate response was to embrace the demands of each pressure group in the union, with the consequence that the 1970 demands were the most extensive ever. On the other side of the negotiating table, the indications were that GM was preparing for a full-scale test of strength with the Reuther leadership in order to tame the union and control labour costs, a strategy that was toned down only when the reins of leadership had passed to Reuther's successor.

There is evidence that the Reuther leadership was heartened by much of the militancy of the late 1960s, especially in so far as it focused on qualitative aspects of work and issues of managerial authority and control. In their view, what was needed was that it should be informed by a wider social and political awareness. Reuther wrote to the Austrian socialist leader Bruno Kreisky in 1968 in worried tones about the growing disintegration of America's social structure:

> I have been much saddened by the fact that the American labor movement has not played the decisive role which it must of necessity play as a creative and constructive force for social change . . . We share the view that the key to the future of the labor movement is the development of young leadership who will have the social idealism and leadership skills necessary . . . to meet new and complex challenges . . .[21]

His solution was to invest heavily in training, not only in leadership but in a form of membership education that also embraced the spouses and children of members. Behind it lay an idealism reminiscent of nineteenth-century Communitarian projects.

In 1965 Reuther had been deeply impressed by a new training school of the Swedish metalworkers' union constructed in a country setting, and inspired by this he obtained authorisation from his own executive board to spend $5 million on a family education centre at Black Lake in the woods of northern Michigan. The Black Lake project became an obsession. It was to be a beautifully constructed education and holiday centre, an example of high craftsmanship, fully equipped with recreational facilities, set in idyllic surroundings, where workers and their families would study the best labour movement and social practices while relaxing in an atmosphere that promoted community ideals and democracy. Reuther took personal charge of the project, and as his frustration in dealings with the AFL–CIO grew, he took solace in the promise of Black Lake, spending more and more time on the site. Meanwhile the construction costs quadrupled and critics began to see him as a megalomaniac engaged in building a shrine to himself. Five modest regionally-based training centres – the proposed alternative to Black Lake – would have been more in keeping with the UAW's spartan traditions. Indeed, the spendthrift nature of Reuther's dream was to become apparent in 1970 when, in the course of a prolonged strike against GM, the union was $10 million in debt and effectively mortgaged to the Teamsters.

Yet the construction of Black Lake was somehow in keeping with Reuther's style in his final years – the project of a restless man, stymied on so many fronts, whose thinking was so much more ambitious than that of his contemporaries. Fittingly, it was to Black Lake that he was travelling by private plane on 9 May 1970 when the aircraft missed the runway at Pellston Airport and crashed into the woods, catching fire. Walter Reuther, his wife, his bodyguard and the Black Lake architect were all killed. Twenty-four years of UAW presidency were brought to an abrupt end. Within a couple of years, the long post-war economic boom that had provided the backdrop to Reutherism would also terminate. An age in the labour movement was rapidly drawing to a close.

8 Reuther in retrospect

Walter Reuther was, arguably, the most important American trade union leader of his generation and one of the commanding figures in the annals of American labour history. In international labour affairs, too, he probably exercised more influence than any contemporary, with the single exception of Jay Lovestone (whose project was of an altogether different and less reputable nature). His early union development took place in the tumultuous years of labour insurgency, while later he became an archetype of the modern labour leader, heading a large, stable organisation operating within the established order. It was easier to cut a heroic figure in the earlier years, and compared with leaders like Eugene V. Debs and Bill Haywood, Reuther led a desk-bound life, though he endured more than his share of violence and was physically very brave. It was, perhaps, also easier for them to retain their professional purity in circumstances where they were excluded from power. However, the trade union world in which Reuther grew to maturity was quite different: he did wield power, inevitably compromises had to be made, and at the same time the skills and talents he was called on to exercise went beyond soap-boxing and the ability to organise a picket line.

He is in some ways a difficult person to assess, for although much has been written about him, and despite the existence of a huge archive of Reuther papers, the fact that he presided over a large organisation that purposely promoted and exploited his fame and prestige can make it hard to evaluate the real Reuther. There was a great deal of highly professional public relations about him. His speeches, writings and ideas were the work of many hands and minds besides his own, and yet he was necessarily the one who took the credit. In reviewing his work, all this has to be taken into account. In a simpler age, Debs and Haywood stood on their own record: Reuther, though a powerful individual, was the front man in a well-organised corporate undertaking.

It was a feature of the Reuther leadership that he surrounded himself with a very able group of committed officers and staff who shared his broad political outlook and philosophy of the labour movement. If 'teamwork in the leadership' was the watchword in the UAW headquarters, the core of that team were Reuther's hand-picked executive assistants and departmental directors, many of whom had been part of his caucus before 1946. A distinctive feature of this group was that they included two of Reuther's three brothers – Victor, who at various times headed the Education Department, the International Department and the union's Washington office, and Roy, whose forte was political organisation. The complex forces at work in family relationships are not easy to divine, and twenty years after his death, when the precise nature of his legacy to the UAW was in dispute, there were open disagreements between Victor Reuther and other former colleagues touching in part on the question of who had been closest to Walter and known his mind best. There was certainly a closeness between Walter and his two younger siblings based on a shared family and ideological tradition, and it seems clear that they complemented each other well. To some it appeared that the UAW leadership was but an extension of the Reuther family, with the brothers at the centre. That is how the brothers sometimes behaved. In fact, Victor and Roy were not Walter's particular confidants: each simply had a job to perform and was in a position to tender advice and contribute to debates, as were all other senior staff. The head office was not heavily structured, but operated more as an informal brains trust, with a natural 'pitching in' where contributions seemed necessary. Though close colleagues, Reuther's circle were not necessarily friends on a personal level: he himself did not socialise with union people and rarely invited them out to his house.

He was a private person whom few people knew intimately. Lacking the easy ability to mix and socialise – he neither smoked, drank nor used profane language – he was not given to saloon bar camaraderie and was never one for small talk. As Edwin Lahey noted in 1946, he had 'none of the charm of the fallible man who goes through life committing indiscretions'.[1] His brother Victor described him as ascetic in his habits, 'high-strung, aggressive and puritanical, sometimes to the point of intolerance'.[2] There was an air of moral righteousness about him, and in a gathering he would be apt to deliver a speech rather than converse. The editor of the *Wage Earner* wrote that Reuther had 'a boy scout simplicity and enthusiasm which shines through everything he does'.[3] He was rarely if ever afflicted by self-doubt, and if at times he was uncertain about the immediate issue, he certainly would not be about the general project at hand.

Many union colleagues were devoted to him, but he had few close friends, and in the years after his shooting was inclined to lead a very private family life at his fortified home outside Detroit with his wife – an influential figure in his life – and two daughters. Lacking a strong sense of humour, and with few interests outside work, fellow union officers sometimes found it hard to pass the time with him off the job, though he could be warm and friendly with people he trusted. He read little for pleasure, rarely visited the cinema or theatre and was not interested in sports, though he took a fishing rod with him when travelling in case an opportunity to relax arose. To some he seemed cold and uninterested in people as individuals, but physical impressions differed. 'His eyes can hold more hate in them than in any man I know,' observed one UAW local officer, while Ernest Hoffman quoted a Detroit clergyman: 'Just look at his eyes. There you will see why Reuther is a man of warmth, honesty and complete sincerity.'[4] He lived for his job: a veritable human dynamo with boundless energy, who worked up to sixteen hours a day, ate and slept little and was invariably in a hurry.

With a broad social vision, he was an indefatigable promoter of plans and projects for the betterment of the human condition, leading the action where he was able, but otherwise pressing others to take the initiative. In this he was a practical man rather than a man of theory, and his schemes were often adaptations of other people's thinking. He had a great facility for listening to a suggestion and then reformulating it, considerably improved. The *500 Planes a Day* proposal; his 1949 plan for building 20 million low-priced houses; the idea for the Peace Corps, first advanced in 1956; and most of all his Total Peace Plan of 1950, in which he proposed the tackling of world poverty through the requirement that countries deposit an annual contribution in a special United Nations account, were just a few of his well-publicised schemes, drafted in a bid to dramatise particular problems and rational ways of resolving them. Often the nub of the proposal was an appeal for more co-operation by people within or between countries, based on the pooling of skills and know-how and frequently involving the cor-poratist idea that governments, labour and employers should work together constructively. This particular theme recurred time after time in the course of the nearly 100 occasions on which he appeared to give testimony before congressional inquiries.

In the narrower confines of the American automobile industry, too, Reuther was an early and persistent advocate of an idea that could well have been the salvation of the industry – that American firms should reverse their traditional strategy and build a line of small, economical cars. He first suggested this in 1949 in a UAW publication, *A Motor Car Named Desire*. As foreign imports ate into the American market from the late 1950s, Reuther repeated the theme, and in 1965 held discussions with President Johnson and Robert McNamara in an attempt to persuade the administration to support the collaborative development of an American small car by the big three corporations. Right through to the end of the 1960s Reuther campaigned on this idea, but met only resistance from the firms.

It was very much on the subject of automation that he acquired a reputation as a modern, innovative labour leader. Reuther encountered this development earlier than most union leaders, for by the mid-1950s new technology was already a persistent problem for the UAW. His approach was to welcome automation, while searching for humane ways of applying it. For him, the foremost requirement was that it be accompanied by expansionist economic policies through which new jobs would be created to replace those automated. He was always optimistic that the logic of this position would eventually dawn on governments and employers. When a Ford executive teased him by asking how he was going to collect union dues from machines in an automated factory, Reuther retorted that the main question was how would the company sell its products to those machines.

Of course, as well as eliminating much laborious work, automation also removed the skill factor from other tasks. As a skilled man who delighted in working with his hands, Reuther understood the significance of this without ever doubting the need to embrace new technology. His approach was that the denial of outlets at work for using creative talents – the 'starvation of the inner man', as he put it – had to be compensated for by satisfying the workers' need for creative expression during their leisure hours. Characteristically, at one time he attempted to establish a woodwork shop in Detroit as a centre for creative relaxation for the union's officers.[5] Indirectly, he hoped, union demands such as the guaranteed annual wage would help humanise the work process in as much as they would force employers to act with increased social responsibility, retaining workers displaced by automation and retraining them where necessary. He urged the creation of a tripartite body to collect information on what developments in automation were planned or in progress, to analyse the costs to labour and the means of sharing equally the benefits. And in the mid–sixties, as a member of Lyndon Johnson's Automation Commission, he endeavoured to generate public awareness of the need for a more systematic approach to the human consequences of technological change. Reuther was the archetypal labour leader of his generation for whom automation was synonymous with progress: in the final analysis, modern work processes had to be endured, offset by the reward of increased leisure and creative relaxation.

In his embrace of automation and new technology, he often seemed to be wholly taken in by the notion of efficiency as a desirable and essentially neutral condition. This tendency, of course, had been clearly evident in his lifestyle and writing as a Ford worker completing high school. Commenting on his early years as UAW president, friendly observers Howe and Widick noted a frightening emphasis on efficiency in his pronouncements,[6] while Daniel Bell likened him to H. G. Wells's satirical notion of the 'new Machiavelli' – the man whose root image of the world is of a limitless spectacle of inefficient operation, of millions of people not organised as they should be. 'Temperamentally, Reuther is no rebel,' wrote Bell, 'nor is he an intellectual ... He is primarily in Veblen's sense an engineer. His emphasis is always on efficiency. His criticism of capitalism turns on the tragedy of waste that a loose society entails. In that sense he is not a radical; he is the cold idealist who wishes to create the functional society.'[7] A true product of the Fordist age, he had no sentimental attachment to small-scale industry. The old liberal concept that bigness was evil and that smallness had a natural virtue was, he believed, so much nonsense.

However, his notion of progress was never one-dimensional. Engineering and technical developments needed to be accompanied by advances in the social sciences. In the last months of his life he told a lecture audience of his worry that people were now schooled in technical know-how but deficient in the how, why or what for. And while society misdirected human resources at the top, it wasted them at the bottom through a mixture of inadequate education and unemployment for too many citizens. Science and technology had expanded man's wealth without expanding his wisdom.[8] The deficiency of the education system was a frequent theme of Reuther's. The crisis of American education was a moral crisis, needing a change of values. Without discarding what was best in American individualism, he wanted schools to promote a greater sense of collectivism, thereby pursuing the American revolutionary goal in an industrial context. The American way of life was not to be overthrown, but truly implemented.[9] So he campaigned for more public spending on education, urging higher pay for teachers and compulsory schooling to eighteen rather than sixteen.[10]

At the same time, he was unwilling to sit back and allow employers to monopolise the development of new technology. He cultivated UAW links with the scientific community and encouraged socially useful research. In 1949 Norbert Weiner, the MIT mathematician, had written to Reuther offering to put at the disposal of the UAW his pioneering research on cybernetics if Reuther would promote its social application. Together, the two men set about developing a Labour–Science–Education Association.[11] By the early 1960s, in conjunction with the Federation of American Scientists, Reuther was hoping to create a body whose role would be to channel scientific and technical breakthroughs in ways likely to raise living standards. They were concerned to promote a co-operative relationship between unions and scientists in projects such as the development of small nuclear reactors for developing countries; 'food for peace machinery', co-operative ventures in the field of electronics, and lobbying for an enlarged budget for research on the problems of disarmament.[12] In a letter to a colleague just two days before his death, Reuther wrote: 'Proud as we are of the role played by UAW members in the manufacture of . . . the first manned vehicle to land on the moon, we are no less determined that the skill, knowledge and dedication which can take man to the stars shall now carry mankind to solutions of earth's ancient afflictions of hunger, ignorance and privation.'[13]

As a labour leader Reuther had all the requisite skills. He was a forceful public speaker, a cool negotiator with an iron nerve, great staying power and a highly developed tactical awareness. If opponents complained that UAW democracy was closely managed, his style of leadership was a model of probity, and there was no shortage of rank-and-file respect for 'the red head' whose modest salary was but a third of that paid to George Meany. There was often considerable flair about

the way he approached activities, as for example during the Ford organising drive when he arranged for the reprinting of 200,000 copies of
Upton Sinclair's anti-Ford novel, *The Flivver King*, for distribution
among workers, or when he hired a plane fitted with a public address
system in an attempt to transmit his union message while flying over the
fortress-like River Rouge plant. With total self-confidence in the recti-
tude of his cause, he combined innate idealism with a measure of pragmatism, urging UAW convention delegates to be driven forward by
idealism, but to think with their heads, not with their hearts. He liked
to retain flexibility of manoeuvre, and whether in collective bargaining
or politics was careful never to confuse an opponent with an enemy.
While pragmatism undoubtedly accounts for his durability, some argue
that in politics it led to compromises which, in the end, blunted his
impulse for fundamental change within the system. He ideas were a
blend of elements of the American progressive tradition and European
social democracy, while he regarded himself as a practical radical –
more radical in practice than his European socialist counterparts.

After dropping out of the Socialist Party, and though a firm proponent of government intervention and tripartism, Reuther was careful
never to allow himself to be branded as anti-free enterprise – in effect
tantamount to being anti-American. His line was to declare himself in
favour of free enterprise, but to point out that as long as it failed to live
up to its promise, state intervention was necessary.[14] He was particularly opposed to the export of American free enterprise values to developing countries, urging Kenyan trade unionists in 1960 to be selective in
what they accepted by way of western aid, and to take the technology,
but leave alone the economic and social values that accompanied it.[15] In
testimony before a Presidential Task Force on International Development two months before his death, he said:

> There is a fixation in America on 'free enterprise'. These words, used as a
> talisman, are frequently intoned by our economic pundits as protection
> against all evil. In my opinion, 'free enterprise' thrives best in relatively
> mature and sophisticated societies. Without a literate population, a decent
> infrastructure, a national administration capable of assessing and collecting
> taxes and an equitable distribution of land, 'free enterprise' is nothing more
> than a license for a few to brutally accumulate capital.[16]

At home his instinct was not to support 'big government', but rather
to see a role for government as a clearing house. The democratic plan-

ning that he spent much of his life calling for did not mean more centralised control, but rather the enlargement of areas of individual decision-
making and voluntary co-operation.[17] He did not share the Marxist view
that labour and capital had irreconcilable interests, believing that, given
the will, the two sides could co-operate constructively. Likewise, he
tended to view the state as a neutral agency, sharing the social democratic belief that the levers of state power would respond to the wishes of
those with a majority in the ballot box. So he rejected the concept of
class conflict. Rather than promoting consciousness of class differences,
his aim was to increase awareness of human similarities. Ever optimistic
about the possibility of human development, he was a rational man who
believed in non-violence.

This spirit animated his thinking on international issues. He identified labour's interests with those of the United States, but he was always
pressing for initiatives through which the two blocs in the Cold War
could co-operate, or at least pursue their competition in less dangerous
ways. From the outset he urged the Kennedy administration to negotiate with both the Soviet Union and the Chinese. In the 1950s he had
complained that America was still operating on negative reflexes – still
fighting against something and shaping policies in the images of fears and
hatreds, without a clear idea of what they were fighting for. He believed
the USSR did not intend to resort to nuclear weaponry, and the only way
a nuclear war would begin would be by accident. The Soviet Union had
come to realise they could not defeat capitalism by force of arms, so the
strategy was to concentrate on economic penetration and political subversion. This was where the battle would be won or lost so the real
challenge was on the economic and social front.[18] Aid to the Third
World was where the superpowers should compete, with the recipients
free to choose the system that best suited them. He argued for American
aid to be given to all free nations, whether or not they were aligned to
the United States. 'Totalitarianism may insist upon political conform-
ity,' he declared, 'but the free world must achieve unity in diversity . . .
America must make it clear that we have no desire to remake others in
our image . . '.[19]

His international trade unionism rested on similar assumptions.
There was a major problem of communist attempts to colonise the trade
union movement, but while matching the weight of their propaganda –
his *Selected Papers* were published in twelve language editions, and at one
point he had ambitions to bring out translations in Urdu, Tamil, Malay,

Bengali and Chinese, aiming at a readership in the region of 500 million
– the answer was not to meet the challenge with subversion, but to
outcompete the opposition by demonstrating that democratic organisation and militant activity were the best ways of improving economic and
social conditions. His sharp pointer to the need to transcend purely
national trade unionism and his practical lead in building union structures for dealing with multinational companies were his greatest le-
gacies to the international labour movement.

In collective bargaining with American employers, Reuther's reputation was solidly built on a series of innovative settlements on wages
and fringe benefits in the 1940s and 50s which set a pattern for other
unions to emulate. Over a twenty-five-year period, he presided over a
doubling of the real standard of living of autoworkers. Critics have
sought to diminish his achievements here, arguing that economic gains
during the post-war boom were easy to come by. Speaking at his last
UAW convention, Reuther himself characterised the auto employers as
a 'golden goose': 'no matter how much fat we take off that goose at the
bargaining table, it has the capability of coming back and the next time it
is even fatter.'[20] However, detractors went further and claimed that the
union and the employers were in a cosy relationship that rewarded
union members for their organisation's accommodation to management control. If that was so, it was a strange sort of sweetheart relationship that had caused the loss of more than 100 million man-hours in local
disputes between 1958 and 1970 at GM alone. In that company it had
taken the union thirteen years of struggle to secure its first pension plan,
eighteen years to win something approaching an annual wage – even
eight years to establish basic in-plant smoking privileges. It is true that
Reuther never resolved the tension between the need for organisational
discipline and the rank-and-file pressure to respond swiftly to production changes that intensified the pace of work. However, in that respect
he was no different from other union leaders of his generation. At issue
here was the question of industrial democracy that would challenge his
successors.

Perhaps the truth is that some left-wing critics expected too much
from the UAW. Although it was far more radical than other American
unions, it was not a socialist organisation, and much as Reuther attempted to wield influence in the political field, the union could not be a
substitute for a political party. In circumstances where the United
States labour movement displayed signs of growing conservatism under

a complacent AFL–CIO leadership, Walter Reuther strove hard through exhortation and example to galvanise the movement into more radical effort. One can only speculate on what he might have achieved at home and internationally had he been given the chance to lead the AFL–CIO. It was the misfortune of the American and international labour movement that the opportunity did not arise.

References

Chapter 1

1 Henry M. Christman (ed.), *Walter P. Reuther: Selected Papers*, New York, 1964, p. 45.
2 Transcript of Interview with Leo Hores, November 1972, Victor Reuther Collection, Box 2 (7), Reuther Archives, Wayne State University, Detroit.
3 Victor G. Reuther, *The Brothers Reuther and the Story of the UAW: A Memoir*, Boston, 1976, pp. 53–4.
4 Walter Reuther, 'Rulers or Servants', 13 November 1929, Victor Reuther Collection, Box 2 (9).
5 Beatrice Hansen, *A Political Biography of Walter Reuther: The Record of an Opportunist*, New York, 1987, p. 6.
6 Victor Reuther to Harry Laidler, 29 July 1958, UAW International Affairs Department, 1956–62, Box 30 (4), Reuther Archives.
7 Herbert Harris, *American Labor*, New Haven, Connecticut, 1938, p. 272.
8 Walter Reuther, 'Auto workers' strike', *Student Outlook*, March 1933.
9 Victor Reuther, *The Brothers Reuther*, *op. cit.*, pp. 94, 100, 102.
10 Victor Reuther Statement, 12 May 1958, UAW International Affairs Department, 1956–62, Box 67(15)
11 Victor and Walter Reuther to Maurice Sugar, 20 June 1935, Maurice Sugar Collection, Box 65 (1), Walter Reuther Archives.
12 Victor Reuther, *The Brothers Reuther*, *op. cit.*, pp. 113–14.

Chapter 2

1 Frank Marquart, *An Autoworkers' Journal*, University Park, Pennsylvania, 1975, p. 61.
2 *Ibid.*, p. 66.
3 Roy Reuther to Tucker Smith, 27 October 1934, Victor Reuther Collection, Box 6(12).
4 Maurice Sugar, 'My Meeting With the Reuthers', Sugar Collection Supplement,. Box 1, Folder 'Incidents for a Book to be Published'.
5 Victor Reuther Collection, Box 65(31).
6 Walter Reuther to Tucker Smith, 29 January 1936, Victor Reuther Collection, Box 3(8).
7 Walter Reuther to Tucker Smith, 22 February 1936, Victor Reuther Collection, Box 3 (8).
8 Walter Reuther to Victor and Roy Reuther, 22 April–2 May 1936, reproduced in full in Kevin Boyle, 'Building the vanguard: Walter Reuther and radical politics in 1936', *Labor History* , 30 (3), Summer 1989, pp. 438–48.

9 Frank Boles, 'Walter Reuther and the Kelsey Hayes strike of 1936', *Detroit in Perspective*, 4 (2), Winter 1980, pp. 85–6.
10 Martin Glaberman, 'Reuther in retrospect', *Liberated Guardian*, 3 June 1970.
11 National Labor Relations Board (621), 1937.
12 Adolph Germer to John L. Lewis, 14 April 1937, Victor Reuther Collection, Box 4 (27).
13 Walter Reuther to Victor and Roy Reuther, 22 April–2 May 1936, *op. cit.*
14 *Ibid.*
15 Irving Howe and B. J. Widick, *The UAW and Walter Reuther*, New York, 1949, p. 74.
16 *Daily Worker*, 17 June 1941.
17 Louis Budenz, *Men Without Faces*, New York, 1948, p. 185.
18 Reuther Administratorship – Ganley Notes, 1952, Box 6 (29), Ganley Collection, Reuther Archives.
19 Martin Glaberman, 'A note on Walter Reuther', *Radical America*, 7 (6), November–December 1973, p. 117.
20 Draft Statement by Walter Reuther to Owen White, July 1937, Victor Reuther Collection, Box 4 (11).
21 *Ibid.*
22 Walter Reuther Statement to Unity Caucus, undated, Summer 1937, Victor Reuther Collection, Box 4 (22).
23 *Ibid.*
24 Transcript of Interview with Jay Lovestone, 23 February 1968, Cormier and Eaton Collection, Box 2 (26), Reuther Archives.
25 Homer Martin Testimony to House Un-American Activities Committee, 1938, p. 2692.
26 *Conveyor*, 17 August 1937.
27 Adolph Germer to John L. Lewis, 30 October 1937, Victor Reuther Collection, Box 4 (22).
28 Harvey Klehr, 'American communism and the United Auto Workers: new evidence on an old controversy', *Labor History*, 24 (3), Summer 1983, pp. 408–9.
29 *Ibid.*, pp. 410–11.
30 Marquart, *op. cit.*, pp. 83–4.
31 'The auto union struggle', *Socialist Call*, 23 July 1938.

Chapter 3

1 'The tradition of Reutherism: interview with Brendan Sexton', *Dissent*, 19, 1972, pp. 57–8.
2 Victor Reuther, *The Brothers Reuther*, *op. cit.*, p. 223.
3 Walter Reuther, *500 Planes a Day: A Program for the Utilisation of the Auto Industry for Mass Production of Defence Planes*, Detroit, 23 December 1940.
4 *New York Times*, 23 January 1941.
5 James Wechsler, 'Labour's bright young man', *Harper's Magazine*, March 1948, p. 267.
6 John Bugas to J. Edgar Hoover, 9 September 1941; J. Edgar Hoover to John Bugas, 1 November 1941. FBI files released under Freedom of Information Act.
7 *Detroit News*, 14 May 1943.

8 Victor Reuther, 'Labor and the War', September 1943, Victor Reuther Collection, Box 19 (24).
9 Walter Reuther and Brendan Sexton, *Are War Plants Expendable?*, Ypsilanti, 1945.
10 Walter Reuther, 'A Wage and Price Program for Conversion', paper for Special CIO Executive Board Meeting, 24 May 1945, Victor Reuther Collection, Box 8 (19).
11 Jean Gould and Lorena Hickock, *Walter Reuther: Labor's Rugged Individualist*, New York, 1972, p. 234.
12 Howe and Widick, *op. cit.*, p. 145.
13 *Life*, 26 November 1945.

Chapter 4

1 'Memorandum on Existing Situation in the International Union', 23 May 1946, Maurice Sugar Collection, Box 1.
2 Ernest L. Hoffman, 'Structural Determinants and the Leadership Role of Walter Reuther in the UAW–CIO', unpublished MA thesis, University of Illinois, Urbana, 1954, pp. 68–9.
3 UAW International Executive Board Minutes, 17–26 March 1947.
4 Bert Cochran, *Labor and Communism: The Conflict that Shaped American Unions*, Princeton, New Jersey, 1979, p. 264.
5 John Herling to Walter Reuther, 31 May 1961, Victor Reuther Collection, Box 29 (6).
6 Frank Cormier and William Eaton, *Reuther*, Englewood Cliffs, N.J., 1970, p. 257.
7 *Convention Proceedings*, UAW, 9 November 1947, p. 8.
8 Report of President to UAW Convention, November 1947, p. 44.
9 Frank Winn to Cormier and Eaton, 28 May 1970, Victor Reuther Collection, Box 70 (28).
10 Jack W. Skeels, 'The Development of Political Stability Within the United Auto Workers' Union', unpublished Ph.D. thesis, University of Wisconsin, 1957, pp. 259–60.
11 Cochran, *op. cit.*, p. 259.
12 Howe and Widick, *op. cit.*, p. 289.
13 Selig Harrison, 'The Political Program of the United Auto Workers', unpublished B.A. thesis, Harvard University, 1948, Introduction.
14 Nelson Lichtenstein, 'Auto worker militancy and the structure of factory life 1937–55', *Journal of American History*, LXVII, September 1980, pp. 349–50, 52.
15 Victor Reuther, *The Brothers Reuther*, *op. cit.*, p. 281.
16 UAW International Executive Board Minutes, 13–15 September 1948, p. 331.
17 UAW International Executive Board Minutes, 28 April 1949, pp. 92–5.
18 Nelson Lichtenstein, 'What happened to the UAW?', *New Politics*, 1 (4), Fall 1976, pp. 36, 39.
19 UAW International Executive Board Minutes, 6–10 June 1949, p. 48.
20 Martin Halpern, 'The Disintegration of the Left-Center Coalition in the UAW, 1945–50', unpublished PhD thesis, University of Michigan, 1982, p. 510.

21 Roy Reuther to Walter Reuther, 16 November 1944, Victor Reuther Collection, Box 79 (2).
22 *Labor Action*, 15 July 1946.
23 Nelson Lichtenstein, 'UAW bargaining strategy and shop floor conflict 1946–70', *Industrial Relations*, 24 (3), Fall 1985, p. 364.
24 Walter Reuther Speech to ADA Conference, Philadelphia, 22 February 1948, cited in Harrison, *op. cit.*, pp. 35–6.
25 *Detroit Free Press*, 4 April 1948.
26 *United Automobile Worker*, April 1948, p. 2.
27 *Ibid.*, August 1948, p. 7.
28 Harrison, *op. cit.*, p. 160.
29 A. H. Raskin, 'Reuther explains the Reuther plan', *New York Times Magazine*, 20 March 1949.
30 *Convention Proceedings*, UAW, 1951, pp. 14–15.
31 *Convention Proceedings*, CIO, October 1947, p. 285.
32 *Convention Proceedings*, CIO, November 1949, p. 266.
33 Roger Keeran, 'The communists and UAW factionalism 1937–39', *Michigan History*, Summer 1976, p. 135; Nelson Lichtenstein, 'Walter Reuther and the rise of labor-liberalism' in M. Dubofsky and W. Van Tine (eds.), *American Labor Leaders*, Champaign, Illinois, 1986, p. 293.
34 Harrison, *op. cit.*, Introduction; Cochran, *op. cit.*, p. 257.

Chapter 5

1 Victor Reuther, *The Brothers Reuther*, *op. cit.*, p. 259.
2 Henry Christman (ed.), *Walter P. Reuther: Selected Papers*, *op. cit.*, pp. 45, 47.
3 *Convention Proceedings*, UAW, 1957, pp 11, 171.
4 Michael Ross to Jay Krane, 29 November 1956, Jay Krane Collection, Box 17 (8), Reuther Archives.
5 Lichtenstein, 'Walter Reuther and the rise of labor-liberalism', *op. cit.*, p. 293.
6 Nat Weinberg to Walter Reuther, 12 June 1950, Weinberg Collection, Box 20, Chronological File May–August 1950, Reuther Archives.
7 Walter Reuther, 'Practical aims and purposes of American labor', *Annals of the American Academy of Political and Social Sciences*, March 1951, p. 71.
8 Report to Membership, *United Automobile Worker*, March 1953.
9 Hoffman, *op. cit.*, p. 175.
10 'The American Auto Workers' Struggle for the Guaranteed Wage', UAW International Affairs Department, 1956–62, Box 116 (13).
11 Lichtenstein, 'UAW bargaining strategy', *op. cit.*, p. 369.
12 Walter Reuther letter to members of US Senate and House of Representatives, 11 January 1957, Weinberg Collection, Box 10, Chronological File January–April 1957.
13 'Policies for Economic Growth; Testimony Presented on Behalf of the American Federation of Labor and Congress of Industrial Organizations to the Joint Economic Committee of Congress by Walter Reuther, Chairman of the AFL–CIO Economic Policy Committee on 9 February 1959', AFL–CIO pamphlet no 8, 1959.
14 Walter Reuther, Speech to SANE Rally, Madison Square Gardens, 19 May 1960, UAW International Affairs Department, 1956–62, Box 32(6).

15 Walter Reuther, 'The United Automobile Workers: past, present and future', *Virginia Law Review*, 50: 58, January 1964, p. 72.

16 'Trade unions without socialism: Walter Reuther talks about American labour to Henry Brandon', part 2, *Sunday Times*, 29 June 1958.

17 'What's wrong with profit sharing plans?', 22 March 1949, Weinberg Collection, Box 20, Chronological File January–June 1949.

18 Walter Reuther to Harlow Curtice, 14 February 1958, Victor Reuther Collection, Box 25 (15).

19 Frank Marquart, 'The auto worker', *Dissent*, IV, Summer 1957, pp. 221–3, 232.

20 B. J. Widick, 'The UAW: limitations of unionism', *Dissent*, Autumn 1959, p. 453.

21 Walter Reuther, 'How Labor and Management Can Cooperate to Preserve Freedom Around the World', Speech to Detroit Economic Club, 30 November 1953.

22 'The tradition of Reutherism: interview with Sexton', *op cit.*, p. 55; Nat Weinberg to Leonard Woodcock, 25 May 1972, Weinberg Collection, Box 15, Personal Correspondence, 1968–72.

23 'Trade unions without socialism: Walter Reuther talks about American labour to Henry Brandon', Part 1, *Sunday Times*, 22 June 1958.

24 A. H. Belmont to L. V. Boardman, 3 March 1958; D. M. Ladd to J. Edgar Hoover, 27 February 1953; J. Edgar Hoover to Tolson, 17 June 1953; A. H. Belmont to D. M. Ladd, 4 June 1953; A. H. Belmont to L. V. Boardman, 17 November 1954. FBI files released under Freedom of Information Act.

25 'Digest of Communist Activities', 29 October 1956, FBI files released under Freedom of Information Act.

26 Senator Barry Goldwater, speech to Detroit Economic Club, 20 January 1958.

27 Senator McClellan to Hubert Humphrey, 16 August 1958, UAW International Affairs Department 1956–62, Box 69(15).

28 *Washington Post*, 28 March 1958, 30 March 1958.

29 Statement by Senator John F. Kennedy, 9 September 1959, Victor Reuther Collection, Box 19 (17).

30 Anthony Carew, *Labour Under the Marshall Plan: The Politics of Productivity and the Marketing of Management Science*, Manchester, 1987, pp. 119–21.

31 Tom Braden, 'I'm Glad the CIA is Immoral', *Saturday Evening Post*, 20 May 1967.

32 Victor Reuther, *The Brothers Reuther*, *op. cit.*, pp. 424–5.

33 Victor Reuther to Walter Reuther, 9 December 1948, cited in Denis MacShane, *International Labour and the Origins of the Cold War*, Clarendon, 1992, p. 139.

34 Walter Reuther to Arne Geijer, 26 May 1959, Victor Reuther Collection, Box 26 (6); UAW International Affairs Department, 1956–62, Box 5 (9).

35 Walter Reuther to Arne Geijer, 22 July 1959, Victor Reuther Collection, Box 26 (11).

36 Konrad Ilg to Walter Reuther, 8 December 1946, cited in MacShane, *op. cit.*

37 Arnold Steinbach, Draft History of the IMF, 1958, pp. 58–63, 118, UAW International Affairs Department, 1956–62, Box 121 (6).

38 *Ibid.*, pp. 70–71: Charles Levinson, Assistance Programme to France/Italy,

papers for IMF Central Committee, 19–24 October 1959, UAW International Affairs Department, 1956–62, Box 113.

39 Victor Reuther to Italo Viglianesi, 9 January 1957, UAW International Affairs Department, 1956–62, Box 2 (9).

40 David Burgess to Walter Reuther, 1 July 1956, UAW International Affairs Department, 1956–62, Box 104 (28).

41 *Sunday Times*, 8 September 1957; *Daily Herald*, *Daily Express*, *News Chronicle* 4 September 1957; 'TUC in conference', *Socialist Digest*, October 1957, p. 5.

42 'Memorandum of Conversation At Luncheon With Soviet Deputy Premier A. I. Mikoyan', 6 January 1959, UAW International Affairs Department, 1956–62, Box 100 (7).

43 John Herling, 'US labor vs. Mikoyan', *New Leader*, 2 February 1959.

44 'Khrushchev and the American unions', The Freedom Fund, April 1960, UAW International Affairs Department, 1956–62, Box 100 (8).

45 *Trud*, 29 October 1959.

46 Arthur Schlesinger, *A Thousand Days: John F. Kennedy in the White House*, New York, 1965, p. 338.

Chapter 6

1 Theodore Sorensen, *Kennedy*, New York, 1965, p. 439.

2 Weinberg memorandum to Walter Reuther, 'Growth, Galbraith and the Election', 1 August 1960, Weinberg Collection, Box 22, Chronological File July–December 1960.

3 *US News and World Report*, 11 March 1963.

4 Cormier and Eaton, *op. cit.*, p. 396.

5 Harvey Swados, 'The UAW – over the top or over the hill', *Dissent*, 10 (4), Fall 1963, p. 338; Lichtenstein, 'Walter Reuther and the rise of labor-liberalism', *op. cit.*, pp. 297–8; Michael Whitty, 'Emil Mazey: Radical as Liberal: the Evolution of Labour Radicalism in the UAW', unpublished Ph.D. thesis, Syracuse University, 1969, p. 241.

6 Victor Reuther to Martin Luther King, 6 August 1963, UAW International Affairs Department, 1962–8, Box 1 (32).

7 'Remarks of Walter Reuther at the 28 August 1963 March on Washington Rally', Victor Reuther Collection, Box 28 (3).

8 Victor Reuther, *The Brothers Reuther*, *op. cit.*, p. 447.

9 Interview with Joseph Rauh, 7 July 1987.

10 Lichtenstein, 'Walter Reuther and the rise of labor-liberalism', *op. cit.*, pp. 297–8.

11 *Detroit Free Press*, 21 June 1964.

12 Lichtenstein, 'UAW bargaining strategy', *op. cit.*, p. 372.

13 Nat Weinberg to Walter Reuther, 5 November 1964, Weinberg Collection, Box 19, Chronological File July–December 1964.

14 Walter Reuther, Statement to Members of President's Advisory Committee on Labor–Management Policy, Weinberg Collection, Box 14, Chronological File June–December 1966.

15 Walter Reuther to Charles Millard, 27 April 1961, UAW International Affairs Department, 1956–62, Box 6 (24); Gould and Hickock, *op. cit.*, p. 332.

16 Walter Reuther to Arne Geijer, 28 January 1960, UAW International Affairs

Department, 1956–62, Box 123 (12); Personal Notes Dictated by Walter Reuther: Separate AFL–CIO Activities in Africa, 3 March 1961, Victor Reuther Collection, Box 31 (11).

17 Walter Reuther to George Meany, 22 June 1961, Victor Reuther Collection, Box 27 (9).

18 Victor Reuther to Walter Reuther, 1 June 1962, UAW International Affairs Department, 1956–62, Box 20 (11); Victor Reuther to Walter Reuther, 2 November 1962, UAW International Affairs Department, 1956–62, Box 7 (36).

19 Victor Reuther to Walter Reuther, 29 July 1964, UAW International Affairs Department, 1962–8, Box 3 (6).

20 A. H. Raskin, 'Walter Reuther's great big union', Atlantic Monthly, October 1963, pp. 86, 92.

21 John Herling, 'Reuther must move', Washington Daily News, 12 September 1961.

22 Convention Proceedings, UAW, 1962, p. 57.

23 Jake Clayman to Walter Reuther, 11 June 1962, UAW International Affairs Department, 1956–62, Box 83 (18); Brendan Sexton and Nat Weinberg to Walter Reuther, 21 January 1963, Weinberg Collection, Box 19, Chronological File January–June 1963.

24 Adolph Sturmthal to Walter Reuther, 7 July 1961; Victor Reuther to Walter Reuther, 21 July 1961, UAW International Affairs Department, 1956–62, Box 40 (22) and Box 6 (30).

25 Willy Brandt to Walter Reuther, 7 January 1963, Victor Reuther Collection, Box 27 (24); Walter Reuther to Willy Brandt, 3 April 1963, Victor Reuther Collection, Box 27 (26); Walter Reuther Note: Follow Thru Per Conversation With Willy Brandt, 11 July 1962, Walter Reuther Collection, Box 463 (5), Walter Reuther Archives.

26 Harold Wilson to Walter Reuther, 29 August 1963; Willy Brandt to Walter Reuther, 15 July 1963; Walter Reuther to Tage Erlander 22 July 1963, Victor Reuther Collection, Boxes 35 (11), 27 (28) and 28 (1).

27 Nat Weinberg to Walter Reuther, 21 July 1965, Weinberg Collection, Box 19, Chronological File July–December 1965.

28 Carl Solberg, Hubert Humphrey: A Biography, New York, 1984, p. 220.

29 Nat Weinberg to Walter Reuther, 3 June 1964, Weinberg Collection, Box 19, Chronological File January–June 1964.

30 Willy Brandt to Walter Reuther, 19 November 1964, UAW International Affairs Department, 1962–8, Box 25 (16).

31 Walter Reuther to Harold Wilson, 3 December 1964, UAW International Affairs Department, 1962–8, Box 25 (16).

32 Walter Reuther to Bruno Storti, 6 June 1962, UAW International Affairs Department, 1956–62, Box 10 (8).

33 Walter Reuther to Italo Viglianesi, 16 June 1961 and Victor Reuther to Corrado de Luca, 4 August 1961, UAW International Affairs Department, 1956–62, Box 6 (27) and Box 7 (2); Victor Reuther, The Brothers Reuther, op. cit., p. 352.

34 Victor Reuther to Italo Viglianesi, 29 May 1962, UAW International Affairs Department, 1956–62, Box 7 (25).

35 Adolph Graedel to Victor Reuther, 8 February 1971, UAW International Affairs Department, 1968–72, Box 39 (19); Victor Reuther to Frank Rosenblum, 18 June 1963, UAW International Affairs Department, 1962–8, Box 1 (25).

36 Fabio Cavazza to Victor Reuther, 12 July 1963, UAW International Affairs Department, 1962–8, Box 35 (20).

37 Adolph Graedel to Walter Reuther, 21 March 1966, Victor Reuther Collection, Box 36 (25).

38 Victor Reuther to Walter Reuther, 7 April 1966, Victor Reuther Collection, Box 36 (25).

39 Minutes of IMF Automotive Conference, Paris, 18 May 1956, p. 5, UAW International Affairs Department, 1956–62, Box 116 (10); IMF Central Committee Minutes, 11–13 September 1963, UAW International Affairs Department, 1962–8, Box 51 (19).

40 Ernest Breech, speech to Pittsburgh Chamber of Commerce, UAW International Affairs Department, 1956–62, Box 93 (21).

41 Walter Reuther, Statement on Foreign Aid to Presidential Task Force on International Development, undated 1970, UAW International Affairs Department, 1968–72, Box 20 (21).

42 Walter Reuther to Omer Becu, 19 June 1961; Walter Reuther to Haruo Wada, 1 February 1962; Joint Statement by Japanese Joint Trade Union Sponsoring Committee and UAW, 24 November 1962, UAW International Affairs Department, 1956–62, Boxes 6 (27), 7 (17) and 108 (7).

43 Victor Reuther to Miyoji Ochiai, 21 October 1963; Stanley Greenspan to Victor Reuther, 13 December 1965; Miyoji Ochiai to Victor Reuther, 26 September 1967, UAW International Affairs Department, 1962–8, Boxes 2 (8), 47 (2) and 58 (16): Memo dictated by Walter Reuther, 'International Wage Research Center', 20 July 1964, Victor Reuther Collection, Box 31 (11).

44 Draft document, 17 October 1960 and Draft Letter to UAW Officers, undated, UAW International Affairs Department, 1956–62, Boxes 118 (1) and 9 (7).

45 Walter Reuther, 'Mobilize the unions against the "super corporations"', Tribune, 6 June 1969.

46 Walter Reuther to Arne Geijer, 17 June 1966, Victor Reuther Collection, Box 28 (10).

47 Transcript of Interview with Jack Conway, 27 December 1967, Cormier and Eaton Collection, Box 2 (11).

Chapter 7

1 Lichtenstein, 'Walter Reuther and the rise of labor-liberalism', op. cit., p. 299.

2 Rauh Interview, op. cit.

3 Walter Reuther to President Johnson, 1 November 1968, Victor Reuther Collection, Box 28 (13).

4 Interview with Irving Bluestone, 17 July 1987.

5 David Halberstam, The Reckoning, New York, 1986, pp. 347–8; Elisabeth Reuther Dickmeyer, Reuther: A Daughter Strikes, Southfield, Michigan, 1989, p. 316.

6 Cormier and Eaton, op. cit., p. 422.

7 'Post Vietnam industrial conversion plan offered', *Journal of Commerce*, 2 December 1969.
8 Martin Glaberman, 'Reuther in retrospect', *Liberated Guardian*, 3 June 1970.
9 Robert H. Zieger, *American Workers, American Unions, 1920–85*, Baltimore, 1986, p. 180.
10 S. Agonistes, 'Reuther puts the brakes on UAW militancy', *Progressive Labor*, VI, June–August 1967, pp. 81–2.
11 *Convention Proceedings*, UAW, 1962, p. 519.
12 'Background of UAW Bargaining', 15 January 1968, UAW International Affairs Department, 1962–8, Box 25 (7).
13 *Factory*, April 1967.
14 Interview with Frank Winn, April 1987.
15 *To Clear the Record: AFL–CIO Executive Committee Report on the Disaffilition of the UAW*, 1969; Transcript of George Meany Press Conference, 13 May 1968, UAW International Affairs Department, 1962–8, Box 38 (24).
16 UAW International Executive Board Minutes, 17 December 1969.
17 Walter Reuther to Petrovic, December 1968, UAW International Affairs Department, 1962–8, Box 40 (9).
18 Victor Reuther, *The Brothers Reuther, op. cit.*, p. 380.
19 Rauh Interview, *op. cit.*
20 Gould and Hickock, *op. cit.*, p. 380.
21 Walter Reuther to Bruno Kreisky, 14 June 1968, Victor Reuther Collection, Box 28 (12).

Chapter 8

1 'Reuther takes over', *New Republic*, 114, 8 April 1946.
2 Victor Reuther, *The Brothers Reuther, op. cit.*, p. 433.
3 *Wage Earner*, 29 March 1946.
4 Hoffman, *op. cit.*, p. 200.
5 *Detroit Free Press*, 5 December 1952.
6 Howe and Widick, *op. cit*, p. 200.
7 Daniel Bell, 'Labour's new men of power', *Fortune*, June 1953, pp. 148–9.
8 Eighth Annual Bronfman Lecture, quoted in *American Journal of Public Health*, 50 (1), January 1969, p. 13.
9 Catherine Valdez, 'Conflict Versus Communication: The Social Philosophy of Walter P. Reuther', unpublished PhD thesis, Fordham University, 1973, pp. 100, 145.
10 Walter H. Slack, 'Walter Reuther: A Study of Ideas', unpublished PhD. thesis, University of Iowa, 1965, p. 146.
11 Norbert Weiner to Walter Reuther, 13 August 1949 and 25 April 1950, Weinberg Collection, Box 20, Chronological Files June–December 1949 and January–June 1950.
12 Victor Reuther to Walter Reuther, 19 March 1962; Lewis Carliner to Victor Reuther, 11 May 1962, UAW International Affairs Department, 1956–62, Boxes 7 (20) and 10 (6).
13 Walter Reuther to Leon Keyserling, 7 May 1970, Victor Reuther Collection, Box 28 (17).

14 Walter Reuther, Testimony to the Senate Committee on Education and Labor, 21 February 1947.

15 Walter Reuther, Speech at Dedication of Kenyan Trade Union Headquarters, May 1960, UAW International Affairs Department, 1956–62, Box 8 (27).

16 Walter Reuther, Statement on Foreign Aid for Presidential Task Force on International Development, op. cit.

17 Walter Reuther, Statement on the Economic Report of the President, 1963, p. 37.

18 'Trade unions without socialism: Walter Reuther talks about American labour', op. cit., Part 2, 29 June 1958.

19 Walter Reuther, 'Report on Asia', UAW International Affairs Department, 1956–62, Box 105 (17).

20 Victor Reuther, The Brothers Reuther, op. cit., p. 305.

Bibliographical Note

The most important source of information on Walter Reuther is the collection of his papers and those of colleagues and fellow union officers at the Walter P. Reuther Archives of Labor and Urban Affairs, Wayne State University, Detroit – the official archive of the United Automobile Workers. Besides Reuther's presidential papers, the most useful collections are the Victor Reuther papers; the UAW International Affairs Department Collection, which includes a considerable body of correspondence between Victor and Walter Reuther, and the Nat Weinberg Collection which casts light on the interaction between Reuther and his principal economic adviser. Also housed at the Reuther Archives are the transcripts of numerous oral histories of UAW officers and activists, many of which deal with aspects of Reuther's rise within the union and his presidency from 1946. Of particular interest are the oral histories of George Addes, Ken Bannon, Jack Conway, Richard Frankensteen, Carl Haessler and Nat Weinberg.

A collection of twenty-one of Reuther's own key writings and speeches appears in Henry M. Christman (ed.), *Walter P. Reuther: Selected Papers*, New York, 1961. Two substantial journal articles by Reuther also deal with his philosophy of the labour movement: 'Practical aims and purposes of American labor', *Annals of the American Academy of Political and Social Sciences*, March 1951, and 'The United Automobile Workers: past present and future', *Virginia Law Review*, January 1964.

Several biographies of Walter Reuther have been written, the first, and in some ways the most perceptive regarding his early politics, being Irving Howe and B. J. Widick, *The UAW and Walter Reuther*, New York, 1949. Eldorus L. Dayton, *Walter Reuther: Autocrat of the Bargaining Table*, New York, 1958 may be regarded as part of the concerted political attack on Reuther by the American right in the late 1950s. Shortly after his death, two journalistic accounts of his life were published, Jean Gould and Lorena Hickock, *Walter Reuther: Labour's Rugged Individualist*, New York, 1972 and a more substantial work by

Frank Cormier and William Eaton, *Reuther*, Englewood Cliffs, 1970. The latter was in preparation at the time of Reuther's death and benefits from extensive interviews with his colleagues and associates. Transcripts of these interviews are to be found in the Cormier and Eaton Collection at the Reuther Archives. Victor Reuther, *The Brothers Reuther and the Story of the UAW: A Memoir*, Boston, 1976 is essentially a first-hand record of the joint activities within the labour movement of Walter and his youngest brother. Inevitably portraying Reuther in a favourable light, it has the virtue of paying more attention to the UAW leader's important international work than do most accounts. John Barnard, *Walter Reuther and the Rise of the Auto Workers*, Boston, 1983 is a more succinct and scholarly treatment of Reuther's career, concentrating largely on his rise to power and his early presidency. Beatrice Hansen, *A Political Biography of Walter Reuther: The Record of an Opportunist*, New York, 1987 is a slim volume arguing the Leninist case against Reuther as a labour leader. Finally, Elisabeth Reuther Dickmeyer, *Reuther: A Daughter Strikes*, Southfield, 1989 is an autobiographical account by Reuther's youngest daughter which reveals details of his home life, of which relatively little is known.

Many sketches of the UAW president from newspapers and magazines are contained in the Biographical File at the Reuther Archives. Among the more perceptive essays on Reuther are James Wechsler, 'Labor's bright young man', *Harper's Magazine*, March 1948; Daniel Bell, 'Labor's new men of power', *Fortune*, June 1953; A. H. Raskin, 'Walter Reuther's great big union', *Atlantic Monthly*, October 1963; 'Walter P. Reuther' in B. J. Widick, *Labor Today: The Triumphs and Failures of Unionism in the United States*, Boston, 1964, and Nelson Lichtenstein, 'Walter Reuther and the rise of labor-liberalism', in M. Dubofsky and W. Van Tine (eds.), *American Labour Leaders*, Champaign, 1986. The latter is of particular note since Lichtenstein has written a series of scholarly articles on aspects of the UAW under Reuther which amount to a sustained critique of the man and the brand of trade unionism that he forged. The companion articles are: 'What happened to the UAW?', *New Politics*, XI (4), Fall 1976; 'Auto worker militancy and the structure of factory life, 1937–1955', *Journal of American History*, September 1980; 'The communist experience in American trade unions', *Industrial Relations*, 19 (2), Spring 1980; 'UAW bargaining strategy and shop-floor conflict: 1946–1970', *Industrial Relations*, 24 (3), Fall 1985, and 'Reutherism on the shop floor:

union strategy and shop-floor conflict in the USA, 1946–1970', in S. Tolliday and J. Zeitlin, *The Automobile Industry and Its Workers*, London, 1986. Lichtenstein's research is thorough, but his many criticisms of Reuther are from a purist position that at times simply fails to recognise the inherent limitations in trade union leadership.

'Reutherism' has often been the subject of university theses, some of which contain valuable insights. Among these are: Selig Harrison, 'The Political Program of the United Auto Workers', B.A. thesis, Harvard University, 1948; George Blackwood, 'The United Automobile Workers of America, 1935–51', Ph.D. thesis, University of Chicago, 1951; Ernest Hoffman, 'Structural Determinants and the Leadership Role of Walter Reuther in the UAW–CIO', M.A. thesis, University of Illinois, 1954; Jack Skeels, 'The Development of Political Stability Within the United Auto Workers' Union', Ph.D. thesis, University of Wisconsin, 1957; Walter Slack, 'Walter Reuther: A Study of Ideas', Ph.D. thesis, University of Iowa, 1965; Catherine Valdez, 'Conflict versus Communication: the Social Philosophy of Walter P. Reuther', Ph.D. thesis, Fordham University, 1973; Arthur Ihrie, 'UAW Convention Speaking, 1955–60', Ph.D. thesis, Wayne State University, 1973, and Martin Halpern, 'The Disintegration of the Left-Center Coalition in the UAW 1945–50', Ph.D. thesis, University of Michigan, 1982

Although there is no comprehensive history of the UAW, many books and articles deal with particular events in which Reuther participated, or with recurrent themes in union politics. Kevin Boyle, 'Building the vanguard: Walter Reuther and radical politics in 1936', *Labor History*, 30 (3), Summer 1989 sheds light on Reuther's politics at the outset of his career as a union leader. Frank Boles, 'Walter Reuther and the Kelsey Hayes strike of 1936', *Detroit in Perspective*, 4 (2), Winter 1980 is an account of Reuther's first major organising success in 1936, while Sidney Fine, *Sit-Down: The General Motors Strike of 1936–1937*, Ann Arbor, 1969 provides a comprehensive account of the union's subsequent confrontation with GM in 1937.

There is an extensive literature on factionalism within the UAW, running from Homer Martin's presidency to Reuther's accession to the top office. Accounts of this are to be found in Walter Galenson, *The CIO Challenge to the AFL*, Cambridge, Mass., 1960; Jack Skeels, 'The background of UAW factionalism', *Labor History*, 2 (2), Spring 1961, and Ray Boryczka, 'Militancy and factionalism in the United Auto

Workers union, 1937–1941', *The Maryland Historian*, 8 (2), Fall 1977. The particular relationship between communism and Reutherism in the factional conflict is best analysed in Bert Cochran, *Labor and Communism: The Conflict that Shaped American Unions*, Princeton, 1979. Other contributions to this debate are Roger Keeran, *The Communist Party and the Auto Workers' Unions*, Bloomington, 1980 and his article, 'The communists and UAW factionalism 1937–39', *Michigan History*, Summer 1976; James Prickett, 'Communism and factionalism in the United Automobile Workers, 1939–1947', *Science and Society*, XXXII, 1968; Harvey Levenstein, *Communism, Anticommunism and the CIO*, Westport, 1981, and Harvey Klehr, 'American communism and the United Auto Workers: new evidence on an old controversy', *Labor History*, 24 (3), Summer 1983. The question of Reuther's possible membership of the Communist Party is discussed in Martin Glaberman, 'A note on Walter Reuther', *Radical America*, 7 (6), November–December 1973.

The effect of the war on UAW politics is considered at length in Nelson Lichtenstein, *Labor's War at Home*, Cambridge 1982, while Martin Glaberman, *Wartime Strikes: The Struggle Against the No-Strike Pledge in the UAW During World War II*, Detroit, 1980 discusses the development of rank-and-file militancy during the war. B. J. Bernstein, 'Walter Reuther and the General Motors strike of 1945–1946', *Michigan History*, 49 (3), September 1965 deals with Reuther's controversial leadership of the strike against GM in 1945–6, and Howell Harris, *The Right to Manage*, Madison, 1982 examines the subsequent reassertion of managerial prerogative through bureaucratic collective bargaining procedures in the late forties.

The nature of the new model unionism developed by Reuther as president has been the subject of many studies. Jack Stieber, *Governing the UAW*, New York, 1962 provides an account of the internal administration of the union during the Reuther presidency. Irving Howe and B. J. Widick, 'The UAW and its leaders', *Virginia Quarterly*, XXV, Winter 1949 is an early piece noting the growing cautiousness of Reuther's leadership. Christopher Johnson, *Maurice Sugar: Law, Labor and the Left in Detroit*, Detroit, 1988, is a friendly biography of one of the leaders of the Addes faction whom Reuther dismissed in 1947. As such, it is highly critical of Reuther's leadership from the days of his first clashes with the communists. Frank Marquart, *An Autoworkers' Journal*, University Park, Pennsylvania, 1975, is a memoir by a one-time Reuther supporter conscious of the growth of bureaucracy in the union. Harvey Swados, 'The UAW – over the top or over the hill?', *Dissent*, X (4), Fall 1963 is one of many contributions which examines the increasing difficulty that Reuther had in mobilising the labour movement in the sixties, while in 'The tradition of Reutherism: an interview with Brendan Sexton', *Dissent*, 19, 1972, a long-time friend and colleague defends the record of Reuther's UAW.

Studies of autoworker collective bargaining have often detailed the way in which the bureaucratic grievance procedure failed to deal with rank-and-file concerns over production standards and related issues. S. Agonistes, 'Reuther puts the brakes on UAW militancy', *Progressive Labor*, VI, June–August 1967 reflects rank-and-file opposition to Reuther's stance on wildcat strikes, while William Serrin, *The Company and the Union*, New York, 1973 is an account of the 1970 collective bargaining round and strike at GM which suggests the existence of a generally cosy relationship between the two sides.

Writers have tended to discuss Reuther's international interests only in passing, and the general subject of AFL–CIO overseas activity has remained a specialism for a handful. My *Labour Under the Marshall Plan*, Manchester, 1987 is an attempt to analyse the contradictory role of American labor in Europe in the Marshall Plan period, highlighting the different objectives of the AFL and the CIO. Henry Berger, 'American labour overseas: Lovestone, Meany and state', *The Nation*, 6 January 1967 and Sidney Lens, 'Labor lieutenants and the Cold War' in Burton Hall (ed.), *Autocracy and Insurgency in Organised Labor*, New Brunswick, 1972 expose the darker side of AFL–CIO foreign policy. John P. Windmuller, 'The foreign policy conflict in American labor', *Political Science Quarterly*, June 1967, gives an account of the growing conflict within the AFL–CIO over the Federation's role in the ICFTU in the 1960s, and Alfred Hero, *The Reuther–Meany Foreign Policy Dispute*, Dobbs Ferry, 1970 provides a detailed account of the issues that divided Reuther and Meany in international policy.

Index

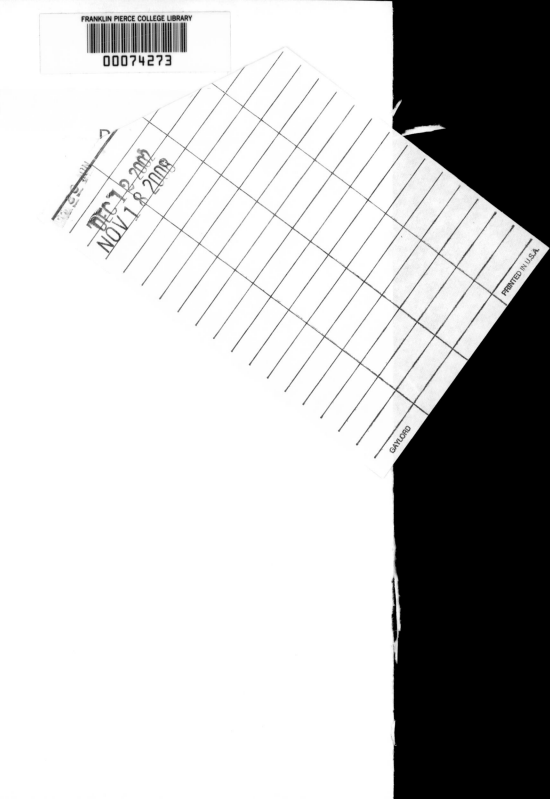